I n 2001, Betty Kitchener and Anthony Jorm developed the Mental Health First Aid Training and Research Program in Australia.

Betty Kitchener and Anthony Jorm have granted permission to the Maryland Department of Health and Mental Hygiene, the Missouri Department of Mental Health and the National Council for Behavioral Health to reproduce and update this copyrighted material for the purposes of improving the mental health knowledge and skills of the U.S. public in responding to early-stage mental illnesses and mental health crises. This manual, which is part of the overall Mental Health First Aid® USA program, was reproduced and updated with funding provided by the Substance Abuse and Mental Health Services Administration Mental Health Transformation State Incentive Grants.

This manual is an accompaniment to the Mental Health First Aid® USA training course designed to teach lay people methods of assisting someone who may be in the early stages of developing a mental health problem or in a mental health crisis. The course information is most relevant in situations where it becomes apparent to others that persons in their social network are developing serious mental health problems. However, the course also may provide useful information on how to assist a person who has a history of a mental disorder or longer-term mental health problems.

The first aid information in this manual is based on guidelines developed by the Australian Mental Health First Aid Training and Research Program from 2006 to 2008, using the consensus of international expert panels involving mental health consumers, caregivers, and professionals. The following people worked on the development of these guidelines: Claire Kelly, Robyn Langlands, Anna Kingston, and Laura Hart. Further details of the guidelines may be found at www.mhfa.com.au.

The content of this publication is informational in nature and is not intended as a substitute for counseling, medical care, peer support, or treatment of any kind.

i

>> Acknowledgments

The Maryland Department of Health and Mental Hygiene, the Missouri Department of Mental Health, and the National Council for Behavioral Health have collaboratively developed the Mental Health First Aid® USA Training Program. First and foremost, we would like to thank Betty Kitchener and Anthony Jorm, founders of the Mental Health First Aid Training and Research Program in Australia. Their guidance throughout this process, countless hours of consultation, and expertise shared in the development of the USA curriculum and program have been extraordinary.

We gratefully acknowledge the many individuals and organizations that contributed to the development of the Mental Health First Aid® USA curriculum. In particular, we would like to thank the following for their vision and invaluable commitment to this program:

- Lea Ann Browning-McNee, Chief Program Officer, Mental Health Association of Maryland

- Carl Clark, MD, CEO, Mental Health Center of Denver and Chair, National Council for Behavioral Health's Board of Directors

- John M. Colmers, Secretary, Maryland Department of Health and Mental Hygiene

- Paolo del Vecchio, Director, Center for Mental Health Services

- Brian Hepburn, MD, Executive Director, Maryland Mental Hygiene Administration

- William Hudock, Special Expert – Financing Policy, Center for Mental Health Services

- Pamela Hyde, Administrator, Substance Abuse and Mental Health Services Administration

- Richard H. Leclerc, President and CEO, Gateway Healthcare and Audit Committee Chair, National Council for Behavioral Health's Board of Directors

- Donald Miskowiec, President and CEO, North Central Behavioral Health System and Member, National Council for Behavioral Health's Board of Directors

- Oscar Morgan, Vice President, Health Management Consultants, LLC

- Joe Parks, MD, Director, Missouri Department of Mental Health Division of Comprehensive Psychiatric Services

- A. Kathryn Power, Regional Administrator, Region One, Substance Abuse and Mental Health Services Administration

- Linda Raines, Chief Executive Officer, Mental Health Association of Maryland

- Keith Schafer, EdD, Director, Missouri Department of Mental Health

- Betty Sims, Missouri Department of Health and Senior Services and former State Senator

- Mark Stringer, Director, Missouri Department of Mental Health Division of Alcohol and Drug Abuse

- The members of the Maryland and Missouri Mental Health, Transformation Working Groups

Among the many organizations that contributed time and resources to this manual, we would like to thank the Anne Arundel County Mental Health Agency, Inc.; Harford County Office on Mental Health; Maryland Coalition of Families for Children's Mental Health; Mental Health America of Eastern Missouri; Mental Health Association of Maryland; Mental Health America of the Heartland, Missouri; Children's Comprehensive System Stakeholder Advisory Group; Missouri Coalition of Community Mental Health Centers; Missouri Foundation for Health; Missouri Institute of Mental Health; NAMI Maryland; NAMI Missouri; On Our Own of Maryland, Inc.; Terezie S. Bohrer & Associates; and the National Council member organizations that piloted the program. These groups worked tirelessly to produce this curriculum and provided valuable comments.

This publication was made possible, in part, by funding through grant number SM57459 to the State of Maryland and grant number SM57474 to the State of Missouri from the Substance Abuse and Mental Health Services Administration (SAMHSA). Its contents are solely the responsibility of the authors and do not necessarily represent the official views of SAMHSA.

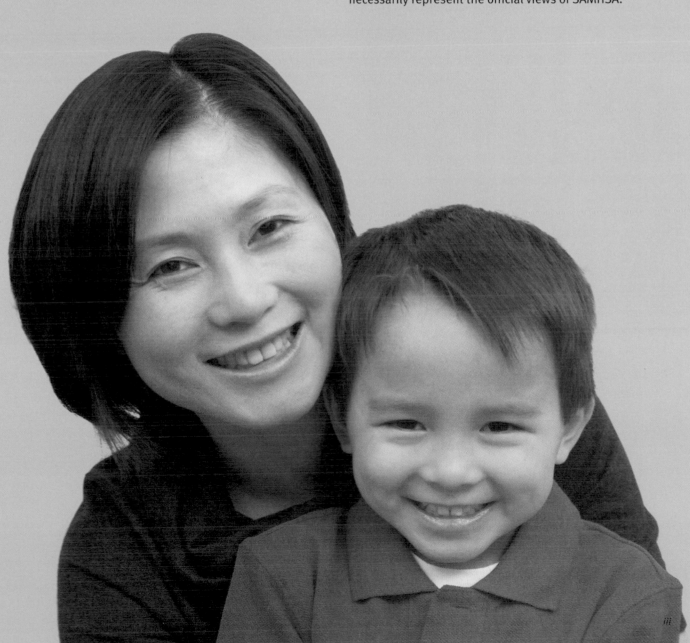

When you think of basic first aid, what comes to mind? Many of us carry first aid kits in our cars, or have taken a basic first aid course. Why? Perhaps we want to be prepared to help a loved one in a medical emergency, or perhaps we have an altruistic desire to be of service if a stranger needs assistance. Knowledge and skills serve us well in navigating an emergency and can potentially *prevent* a medical emergency through early intervention. Mental Health First Aid® (MHFA®) aims to do both: teach members of the public how to respond in a mental health emergency and offer support to someone who appears to be in emotional distress.

The terms *mental illness, mental health,* and *mental disorders* are tossed around freely in today's society, and yet many of us aren't clear about their meanings or relevance to our lives. Most of us assume mental illness is something that only affects others and believe it won't affect our family or friends. The truth is that mental health problems are more common than heart disease, lung disease, and cancer combined.[1, 2]

Mental health issues affect *all* of society in some way, shape, or form. It's estimated that one in five Americans will experience a diagnosable mental disorder in any given year.[3] It is extremely likely you will encounter someone in your family, workplace, school, church, or community who lives with a diagnosed mental disorder. In addition, you will encounter others who are experiencing distress or facing a mental health challenge that may require support and assistance, but not medical intervention.

By using this manual you can acquire the basic knowledge and skills to respond to an individual in distress. To maximize the manual's effectiveness, it is important to understand how the information fits into the larger context. For instance, this manual offers education on signs and symptoms of a variety of diagnosable mental disorders, such as depression, anxiety, substance use, eating disorders, trauma,

psychosis, and deliberate self-injury. It describes, in detail, how you can assist in specific situations. It is oriented toward getting a person appropriate help from a health professional. But it's important to note that while many mental disorders are effectively treated in a professional setting, many mental health problems can be resolved or helped by seeking support, restoring emotional balance, and employing self-care strategies. Just as with physical health, people may use many effective alternative and complementary strategies.

Not every person in psychological distress has a mental disorder. While you may observe someone who seems to match the signs and symptoms listed in the manual for a particular disorder, it doesn't necessarily mean that is the case. The information presented here is designed to help you assume a helpful role when encountering a distressed individual and should not be used to diagnose or to replace a therapist. The strains, stresses, and challenges of today's society increase our vulnerability and likelihood of encountering many mental health problems and mental disorders. Determining where someone falls on the continuum of health/mental health is beyond the scope of this training.

A word of caution: When we gain information or insight into a particular field of study, we often start to see it everywhere, much like the plethora of red convertibles that magically appear on the highways once we've decided to buy one! So as you travel through this MHFA® training, be aware that it's easy to start seeing mental disorders in places they don't exist. Human beings are complex creatures with a wide range of emotions and experiences, and it's important to resist interpreting the common vicissitudes of emotion as pathology.

This manual contains diagnoses and descriptions. However, it is important to distinguish between the person experiencing a mental health crisis and the problem or circumstance itself. It is neither accurate nor fair to define people by their perceived conditions. We believe it warrants mentioning because of the stigma and discrimination associated with mental health. While you would be hard pressed to hear someone referred to as "a cancer," or "a broken leg," we often do hear people referred to as "manic depressives" or "schizophrenics." This kind of derogatory labeling is disrespectful and creates a formidable barrier to recovery.

This Mental Health First Aid® USA (MHFA® USA) manual is a blueprint for providing comfort, promoting recovery, and helping to reduce distress related to stressful situations, trauma, and crisis. Think of it as a guidebook that gives you tools to build a trusting relationship that will help you help others.

Trust and relationship are key concepts here. Many individuals in distress avoid seeking help or are skeptical of those who offer assistance because of the widespread stigma of mental illness. *Stigma* is a cluster of negative attitudes and beliefs that motivate the public to fear, reject, avoid, and discriminate against people with mental illnesses.[4] Stigmatizing attitudes and beliefs about mental illness are common, and the ramifications are serious. Many suffer in silence rather than risk discrimination or ridicule if they seek help. Stigma assumes many forms, subtle and overt, and can negatively affect all areas of life—housing, employment, and, certainly, relationships. Stigma can appear as prejudice, discrimination, fear, distrust, and stereotyping. Stigma not only may prevent people from seeking help—it may prevent them from acknowledging they need help. Stigma may affect access to care and quality of care and, perhaps worst of all, may result in the person internalizing negative attitudes about himself or herself.

> "The last great stigma of the twentieth century is the stigma of mental illness."
> — TIPPER GORE

Stigma is one of the biggest barriers to individuals seeking treatment, and therefore is one of the biggest barriers to recovery.[115] Fighting the stigma and shame associated with mental illness is often more difficult than battling the illness itself.

> "Mental illness is nothing to be ashamed of, but stigma and bias shame us all."
> — FORMER PRESIDENT BILL CLINTON

That shame has far-reaching effects. The person you try to help might deny a problem or refuse help because of stigma. Or they might distrust your motives, fearing you might harbor stigmatizing or discriminatory thoughts. In fact, you may. This MHFA® USA manual will help you examine your own ideas about mental health and mental illness. None of us grows up in a vacuum—we grow up surrounded by the attitudes of family and friends, and we often are influenced in ways we don't even realize until we find ourselves in situations where we confront those preconceived ideas. What would happen if you found out someone close to you had a diagnosable mental health problem? Would it change your opinion of that person? Would it cause you to question his or her judgment? Would you find yourself being less than honest or "walking on eggshells" when talking to him or her?

> "Where I worked, if you had a heart problem or cancer, you'd never find a more sympathetic, supportive group of people ... but for years I had to be secretive about my mental illness because I was in control of millions of dollars of the corporation's assets, and I couldn't run the risk of having my judgment mistrusted."
> — PAUL GOTTLIEB, PUBLISHING EXECUTIVE

Misconceptions abound regarding mental health issues, and we may have accepted some of those myths without even realizing. Let's take a look.

MENTAL HEALTH, ILLNESS, AND DISORDERS: CHALLENGING MYTHS

Mental disorders were once thought to affect very few, but today we know the opposite is true. Many people with these conditions lead full, productive, and satisfying lives. Despite living with a diagnosis such as substance use disorder, eating disorder, depression, bipolar disorder, or schizophrenia, people go to work, vote, own homes and businesses, and contribute to their communities. Even as negative myths abound, there is hope and renewed optimism regarding the outcomes of living with mental health challenges.

As recently as 20 years ago, people did not dare whisper the word "cancer," as it was considered an automatic death sentence. Yet we now know that many live full lives despite cancer. The same is true for mental illness. It was once a common belief that those with mental illnesses should be locked away in institutions. We now know there are a significant number of people with mental health issues who lead productive lives and enrich our communities. *Good mental health* and *mental illness* are not polar opposites, but points on a continuum. *Good mental health* is a state of successful performance of mental function, resulting in productive activities, fulfilling relationships, and the ability to cope and adapt. It is something we work toward every day. Good mental health includes emotional balance, the capacity to live fully, and the flexibility to deal with life's inevitable stresses, challenges, and trauma. Mental health is very important in terms of personal well-being, family and interpersonal relationships, and meaningful participation in society.

Mental disorders are diagnosable illnesses characterized by alterations in thinking, mood, or behavior (or some combination), which can be associated with distress and, sometimes, the ability to function in daily life.

Common misconceptions include the following:

>> **Mental disorders are signs of weakness or personality flaws. If someone wants to be happy, they simply can be happy. If you ignore the problem and use willpower, the problem will simply go away.**
These beliefs are inaccurate and hurtful. Mental disorders cannot be willed away. Ignoring the problem typically makes it worse. Treatment strategies will differ for each individual, but professional help is the first step. Depression and the other major mental disorders have nothing to do with laziness or lack of willpower.

>> **People with mental disorders are violent.**
Individuals living with mental disorders are no more likely than a member of the general population to commit a violent act. Research shows that as a group, people with mental disorders are far more likely to be victims of violence than perpetrators. More than one quarter of persons with severe mental illness had been victims of a violent crime in the past year, a rate more than 11 times higher than the general population.[5] Put another way, research has shown that the vast majority of people who are violent do not suffer from mental disorders.[6]

>> **"Healthy" people aren't affected by traumatic events. If they are, it's because they really do have a mental health problem.**
Trauma can affect anyone, regardless of how strong or psychologically healthy. As Viktor Frankl, concentration camp survivor and founder of Logotherapy, stated, "An abnormal reaction to an abnormal situation is normal behavior."[7] Current history is marked by staggering progress and unlimited potential; it also is marked by economic turbulence, widespread domestic issues, high rates of violence, and unrest between nations. Many events and situations are considered traumatic and have significant negative physical, social, and emotional impact on people of varying socioeconomic and cultural–ethnic backgrounds. For instance, as military personnel return from Iraq and other war-torn countries, we are seeing astonishing rates of

suicide, [8, 9, 10] indicating a clear and growing need for mental health services to deal with the emotional consequences of war and the emotional strains of wounded soldiers.

It is critical to learn as much as you can to challenge such myths, both in others as well as in yourself. One powerful and accurate lens through which to view mental health problems and disorders is called the *recovery paradigm*.

THE RECOVERY PARADIGM

There is an alternative paradigm for treatment of mental health problems and disorders that embraces the notion of recovery and wellness. Research and experience show that persons living with mental disorders and mental health problems can lead full lives and be contributing members of society.[11, 12, 13] Groundbreaking research in the 1980's by Courtney Harding and associates demonstrated that persons with even severe forms of mental disorders could live productive lives. The researchers followed people 30 years after leaving an institutional setting and found that a high percentage were living successfully in communities *with little or no access to formal mental health services*. No matter how long a person has experienced symptoms of mental illness, or how severe the symptoms appear, people can and often do recover.

Recovery is a deeply personal process of (re)gaining physical, spiritual, mental, and emotional balance. The person learns to cope with illness, crisis, or trauma and its associated challenges while adjusting their lifestyles. Recovery, therefore, is a process of healing and restoring health and wellness during stressful episodes of life.

The President's New Freedom Commission Report defined recovery as "the process in which people are able to live, work, learn, and participate fully in their communities. For some individuals, recovery is the ability to live a fulfilling and productive life despite a disability. For others, recovery implies the reduction or complete remission of symptoms."[4] The federal Substance Abuse and Mental Health Services Administration outlined the following core components of recovery:

HOPE: The most important facet of recovery is hope. It is the catalyst of the recovery process, and without hope, situations involving psychological distress can deteriorate rapidly. When one is in the midst of emotional distress, it can be difficult to hold onto hope that things can change. The role you play in fostering hope may be the most valuable contribution you can make in supporting someone in a mental health crisis.

NONLINEAR: Recovery isn't step by step—it's a nonlinear process. To achieve continual growth, there will be occasional setbacks. This phenomenon isn't unique—it applies to recovering from surgery, trying to quit smoking, getting over the common cold, or even getting past heartache! Realize that backward slides or sideways steps aren't failures, but part of the recovery process.

STRENGTHS-BASED: Focusing on strengths rather than deficits is an integral part of recovery. Particularly during the initial stage of awareness, it is important to view the person as an individual, with unique strengths and challenges. People living with mental disorders feel downgraded by those who concentrate solely on attempting to ameliorate weaknesses or challenges. Rather than viewing the person as a broken entity that needs fixing, the recovery paradigm focuses on valuing and building on strengths, capacities, resiliencies, talents, and inherent worth. Because you may be encountering a person at this initial stage, it is all the more important to realize your actions and reactions can have significant impact. Viewing someone from a strengths-based perspective can enhance self-esteem and cultivate wellness and coping skills.

PEER SUPPORT: Sharing experiences, knowledge, and skills is an important aspect of recovery. Steering a person in distress toward sources of peer support can be a valuable part of Mental Health First Aid®, just as it might help someone battling cancer to find a cancer support group. For people with mental disorders and their families, support groups have been found to be helpful.[14, 15] Support groups can be an important adjunct or alternative to formal mental health treatment. Participation in self-help groups has been shown to reduce feelings of isolation, increase knowledge, and enhance coping skills as well as bolster self-esteem. People establish social networks that prevent isolation, promote health, and reduce the incidence or severity of illness. Support can reduce the stigma associated with mental illness and foster early detection of ill-nesses.[52]

> "The provision of mental health support services by persons who have experienced mental and substance abuse conditions make use of empathy and empowerment to help support and inspire recovery."
>
> — POSITION STATEMENT 37, MENTAL HEALTH AMERICA

SELF-DIRECTION: Recovery is a process that must be directed by the individual, who defines his or her own goals and designs a unique path toward those goals. Recovery is possible when people assume personal responsibility for their own self-care, learn coping strategies, and seek support. The concept of self-direction is important to recognize as you are engaged in the process of giving mental health first aid. Remember, you are not there as an expert—you are there to assist. This would be true even if you were a licensed mental health professional. The person in distress is the one who knows best and who ultimately makes decisions about what to do. Even if that person is incapacitated, supporters should utilize advance directives so that the person's wishes can be carried out in the event he or she is unable to make decisions in a time of crisis.

RESPONSIBILITY: We all must assume responsibility for our own self-care and journey of recovery. Taking steps toward these goals may require great courage. Recovery includes working to understand and give meaning to one's experiences and identify coping strategies and healing processes to promote personal wellness.

HOLISTIC: Recovery encompasses an individual's whole life, including mind, body, spirit, and community. Recovery embraces all aspects of life, including housing, employment, education, mental health and healthcare treatment and services, complementary and naturalistic services, addiction treatment, spirituality, creativity, social networks, community participation, and family support. As you attempt to assist persons in distress, it is important to realize there may be multiple layers affected by their present condition or problem.

INDIVIDUALIZED AND PERSON CENTERED: Each person's vision of recovery and journey of recovery are unique, based on an individual's needs, preferences, experiences (including past trauma), and cultural background. *One size definitely does not fit all.* Some people may need a push, others may need extra support in times of distress, and some may just need a shoulder to lean on. What it means to be mentally healthy is subject to many interpretations rooted in value judgments that may vary across cultures. Thus, reactions to distress and seeking help also have cultural implications. It's helpful to see the situation from the person's unique point of view in order to understand the person's need for and possible response to your caring, support, and guidance.

EMPOWERMENT: The person who is in emotional distress has the right and authority to choose from a range of options and to participate in decisions that affect recovery and wellness.

RESPECT: Crucial to recovery is societal acceptance and appreciation of all persons, including protecting their rights and eliminating discrimination and stigma. Self-acceptance and regaining belief in one's self are particularly vital. Respect ensures inclusion and full participation in all aspects of life.

YOUR ROLE IN MENTAL HEALTH FIRST AID®

It is well known that *social support* plays an important role in helping people to strengthen their ability to cope with stress and adversity. Social support, in addition to coping skills, self-care, and self-esteem, has a powerful impact on lessening the incidence of mental disorders and stress-related illness. The field of public health has a long history of recognizing the powerful influence of bolstering protective factors. Though a person may encounter risk factors, such as biological conditions, exposure to stress, exploitation, and trauma, the strengthening of protective factors can lessen the incidence of illness or disorder. Such factors include coping skills, self-esteem, self-care skills, and social support systems.

When offering mental health first aid, you are the first line of support. You are there to help the person to feel less distressed, and you can be a vital source in helping the person to seek further assistance. Your body language, what you say, and how well you offer a listening ear can have a powerful impact. The quality and type of support you offer through listening can enhance coping and self-esteem. Approaching the person with an accurate view of mental health issues and from a strength-based holistic perspective, you can enhance self-esteem and help him/her to help himself or herself, including cultivating wellness, self-care, and coping skills.

MENTAL HEALTH FIRST AID®: EMPATHIC LISTENING

> "The most basic and powerful way to connect to another person is to listen. Just listen. Perhaps the most important thing we ever give each other is our attention... A loving silence often has far more power to heal and to connect than the most well-intentioned words."
>
> — RACHEL NAOMI REMEN, CLINICAL PROFESSOR OF FAMILY AND COMMUNITY MEDICINE, UNIVERSITY OF CALIFORNIA, SAN FRANCISCO SCHOOL OF MEDICINE

A core aspect of giving mental health first aid is *being fully present and listening*. As human beings, we have a fundamental need to be understood. Not necessarily agreed with, but understood! Being fully present and truly listening can help minimize feelings of distress and may be the most effective link in helping a person to seek support or treatment that fosters personal wellness. The core mental health first aid skills are communication and effective listening. Listening involves *all* of you, not just your ears! The way we are perceived can be based on body language and tone of voice, so it is important to recognize what your nonverbal language is saying. In order to effectively offer MHFA®, it is important that you suspend your judgment or biases.

›› It is critical that you assess your own preconceived notions, attitudes, concerns, and beliefs regarding mental illness in order to effectively offer assistance to someone in need. Allow the person with the problem to do most of the talking.[16]

›› Avoid premature conclusions based on your life experiences.

›› Help the individual to better understand himself or herself.

›› Permit the person to retain ownership of the challenge.

>> Show the person that you are listening without judging.

Another mental health first aid skill is an *optimistic attitude* regarding the outcome of someone in distress. The renewed hope regarding the outcomes of living with mental health problems and mental disorders includes a focus on wellness. The notion of wellness is now considered a core guiding principle for mental health practice.[17] Wellness is a conscious, deliberate process that requires a person to become aware of and make choices for a more satisfying lifestyle.[18] A wellness lifestyle includes a balance of such health habits as adequate sleep, productivity, exercise, participation in meaningful activities, nutrition, social contact, and supportive relationships. Wellness views a person holistically and includes physical, emotional, intellectual, social, environmental, and spiritual dimensions. Significant research reveals the health benefits of physical exercise on mental and emotional well-being. In addition, there is significant research on the value of social support for well-being.[19]

It is important to understand that wellness and recovery are possible and that those who experience mental health problems and disorders can and do lead full lives, often with limited or no professional intervention. People may experience a diagnosable condition due to life's stressors but find resilience and progress to recovery. Mental Health First Aid® is a tool designed to help you gain a better understanding of the signs of someone in distress, offer immediate support to minimize that distress, and if necessary link the person to available professional or self-help support resources. As you proceed through the manual, remember that you play a valuable role in offering support that enhances the wellness of yourself and others.

FOREWORD BY PEGGY SWARBRICK, PhD, AND
JENNIFER K. BROWN, BA

AUGUST 5, 2008

MARGARET (PEGGY) SWARBRICK, PhD, OTR, CPRP, is director of the Institute for Wellness and Recovery Initiatives, Collaborative Support Programs of New Jersey and a part-time clinical assistant professor in the Department of Psychiatric Rehabilitation and Counseling, University of Medicine and Dentistry of New Jersey—School of Health Related Professions. Peggy has been personally involved in the mental health field since 1977 and professionally since 1986. Her experience as a recipient of mental health services inspired her work and passion to advocate for and create services based on wellness, recovery, and peer support. Peggy has authored numerous publications and has lectured nationally and internationally on issues such as wellness, recovery, employment, and peer support.

JENNIFER K. BROWN, BA, has worked in the mental health field since 1994, currently serving as director of training and communications for On Our Own of Maryland, Inc., a statewide consumer advocacy and training organization. She directs the nationally known Anti-Stigma Project, a collaborative education effort that tackles the complex subject of stigma and discrimination associated with mental health issues. She has presented nationally and internationally on issues such as stigma and discrimination, trauma-informed care, culture change, and recovery principles. She specializes in group facilitation, training of trainers, curriculum development and implementation, and video development.

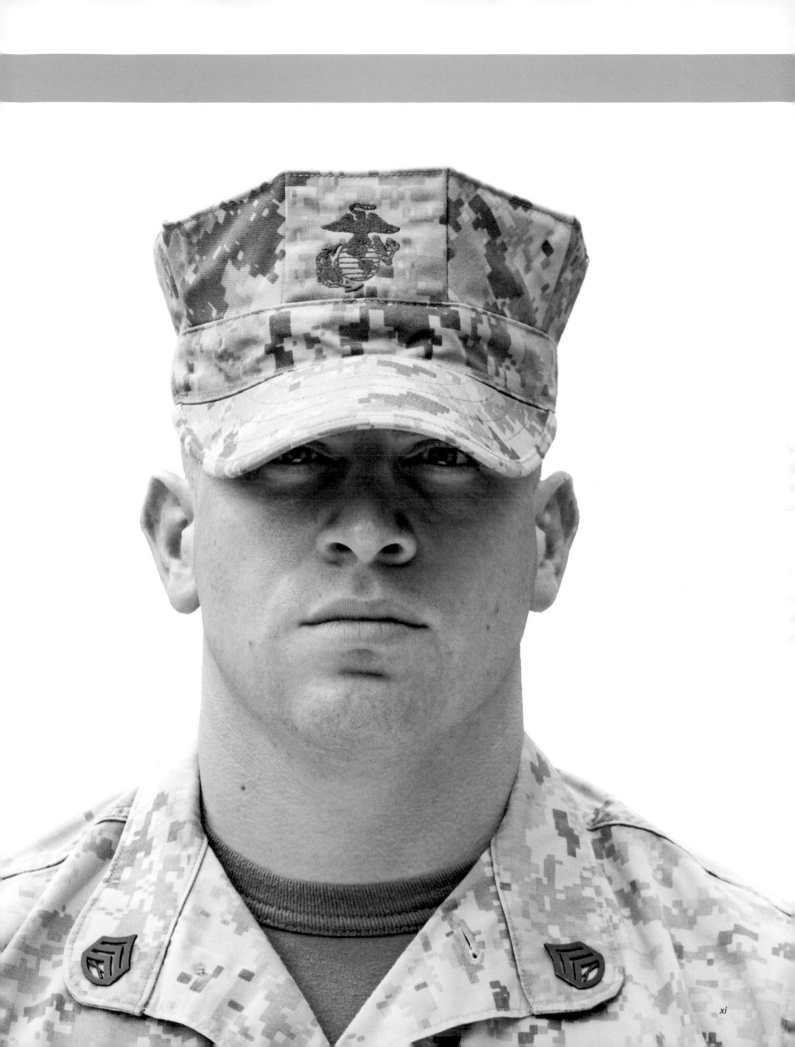

>> Contents

SECTION THREE: FIRST AID FOR MENTAL HEALTH CRISES

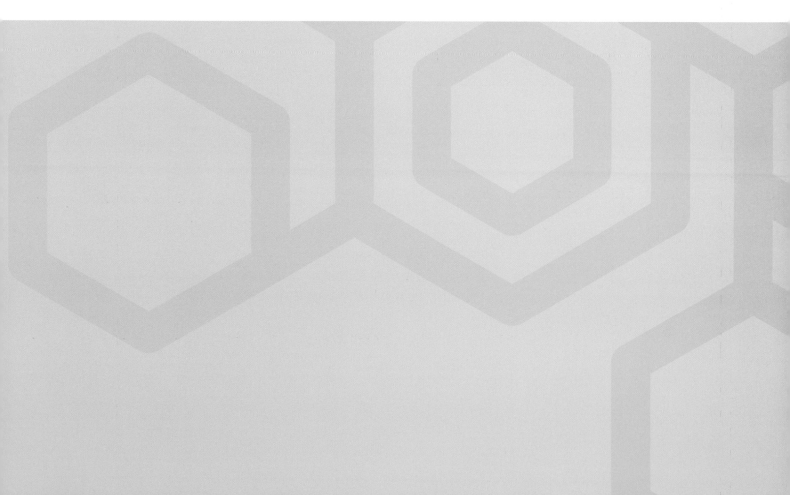

SECTION ONE: Mental Health Problems

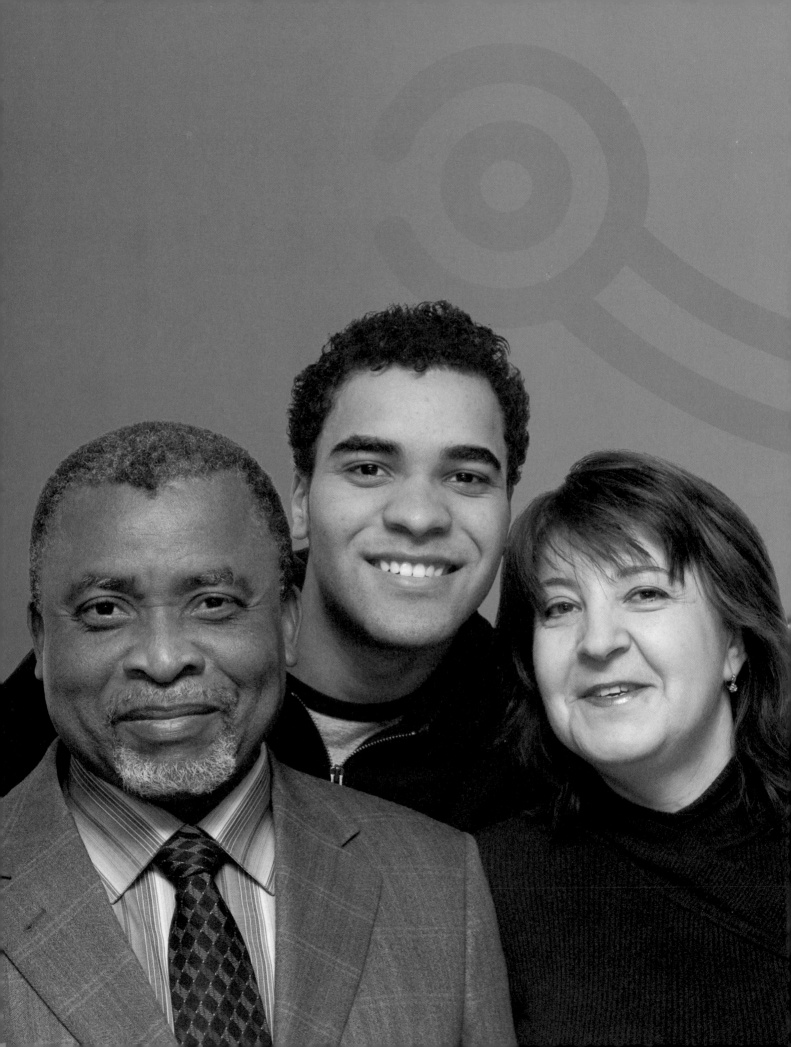

CHAPTER 1

Mental Health Problems in the United States

What Is Mental Health?

There are different ways of defining mental health. Some definitions emphasize positive psychological well-being; others see it as the absence of *mental health* problems.

For example, the World Health Organization has defined mental health as follows: *Mental health can be conceptualized as a state of well-being in which the individual realizes his or her own abilities, can cope with the normal stresses of life, can work productively and fruitfully, and is able to make a contribution to his or her community.*[20]

In this Mental Health First Aid® USA manual, *mental health* is seen as a continuum ranging from having good mental health to having mental disorders. A person will vary along this continuum at different points in his or her life. A person with good mental health will feel in control of their emotions, will have good cognitive functioning, and will have positive interactions with people around him or her. This state allows a person to perform well at work, in their studies, and in family and other social relationships.

What Are Mental Health Problems?

A variety of terms are used to describe mental health problems: *mental disorder, serious emotional disorder, extreme emotional distress, psychiatric illness, mental illness, nervous exhaustion, mental breakdown, nervous breakdown,* and *burnout.* Slang terms include *crazy, psycho, mad, loony, nuts, cracked up,* and *wacko.*

These terms do not give much information about what the person is really experiencing. **A mental disorder** or mental illness is a diagnosable illness[21] that affects a person's thinking, emotional state, and behavior and disrupts the person's ability to work or carry out other daily activities and engage in satisfying personal relationships.

There are different types of mental illnesses, some common, such as depression and anxiety, and some not so common, such as schizophrenia and bipolar disorder. However, mental disorders, as with any health problem, lead to disability, which is sometimes severe. This is a factor not often appreciated by people who have never experienced a mental disorder.

A mental health problem is a broader term that includes both mental disorders and symptoms of mental disorders that may not be severe enough to warrant the diagnosis of a mental disorder.

This Mental Health First Aid® USA manual provides information on how to assist people with mental health problems and not only those with diagnosable mental disorders. There are so many different types of mental health problems that it's not possible to address them all in this manual. Only the most common and most severe problems are included. It is important to note that the first aid principles found in this manual can be usefully applied to other mental health problems.

How Common Are Mental Disorders?

Mental disorders are common in the United States, with one in five adults having a mental disorder in any one year. A national survey of Americans found that 19.6 percent of adults (18 or older) experienced a mental disorder in any one year. This is equivalent to 45.6 million people.[3]

Percentage of American Adults with Mental Disorders in Any One Year	
TYPE OF MENTAL DISORDER	ADULTS
Anxiety disorders	19.1 %[1]
Major depressive disorder	6.8 %[1]
Substance use disorder	8 %[90]
Bipolar disorders	2.8 %[1]
Eating disorders	2.1 %[22]
Schizophrenia	0.45 %[23]
Any mental disorder	19.6 %[3]

This survey, conducted from 2001 to 2003, reflects the entire adult population of the United States. Research on subgroups within the population may show higher or lower rates of mental disorders.

Mental disorders often occur in combination. For example, it is not unusual for a person with an anxiety disorder to also develop depression, or a person who is depressed to misuse alcohol or other drugs, perhaps in an effort to self-medicate. Terms used to describe having more than one mental disorder are *dual diagnosis, comorbidity,* and *co-occurrence.* Of the 26.2 percent of U.S. adults with any mental disorder in a 1-year period, 14.4 percent have one disorder, 5.8 percent have two disorders, and 6.3 percent have three or more.[1]

Impact of Mental Disorders

Mental disorders often start in adolescence or early adulthood. In fact, a national survey reported that half of all mental disorders began by age 14 and three quarters by age 24.[2] When mental disorders start at this stage, they can affect the young person's education, movement into adult occupational roles, forming of key social relationships (including marriage), and establishment of health habits, such as alcohol or other drug use. Consequently, mental disorders can cause disability across a person's lifespan. It is important to detect problems early to ensure the person is properly treated and supported.

Medical experts rate mental disorders among the most disabling illnesses.[24] Often the illness leads to premature death. Disability is the disruption a health problem causes to a person's ability to work, care for himself or herself, and carry on relationships. However, because disability caused by mental disorders may not be visible to others, people with mental disorders can be negatively judged as being weak, lazy, uncooperative, or not really ill. This lack of understanding contributes to the stigma of people with mental disorders. It helps to understand the degree of disability that mental disorders can cause by comparing it to physical illnesses. Some examples:

1. The disability caused by *moderate depression* is similar to the impact from relapsing multiple sclerosis, severe asthma, or chronic hepatitis B.

2. The disability from severe depression is comparable to the disability from quadriplegia.[24]

DISEASE BURDEN IN NORTH AMERICA, 2004[25]

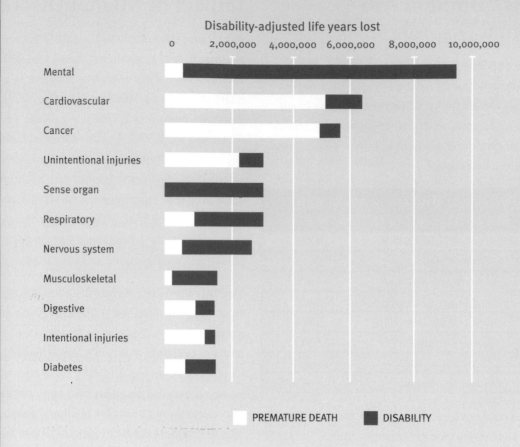

Disability-adjusted life years lost

PREMATURE DEATH   DISABILITY

In recent years, the World Health Organization (WHO) has compared the relative impact of different illnesses across the world on disease burden.[25] *Disease burden* is the combined effect of premature death and years lived with disability caused by illness. According to the WHO data, mental disorders rank as the biggest health problem in North America, ahead of both cardiovascular disease and cancer.[26] Of the different mental disorders, depression is the biggest single cause of disease burden.

Spectrum of Interventions for Mental Health Problems

Society has a wide range of interventions for preventing mental health problems and helping people with mental disorders. Mental Health First Aid® (MHFA®) is just one part of the spectrum of intervention. The following figure shows how a person moves from wellness to developing mental health problems, which may progress to a diagnosable mental disorder and then on to recovery. Different types of interventions are appropriate for these states of mental health. For the person who is well or with mild symptoms, prevention programs are appropriate. For the person who is moving toward a mental disorder, early intervention approaches can be used. For a person who is very unwell with a mental disorder, a range of treatment and support approaches are available to assist the person in the recovery process.

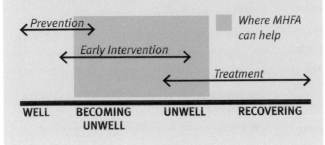

SPECTRUM OF MENTAL HEALTH INTERVENTION SHOWING THE CONTRIBUTION OF MENTAL HEALTH FIRST AID

Prevention

Prevention programs are available to everyone, and targeted programs are for those particularly at risk. These programs can include campaigns to reduce the stigma of mental disorders, drug education programs in schools, resilience training, stress management courses, and parenting skills.

Early Intervention

Early intervention programs target people with mental health problems and those who are developing mental disorders. They aim to prevent problems from becoming more serious and reduce the likelihood of secondary effects such as job loss, school dropout, relationship breakup, and drug and alcohol problems. Many people have a long delay between developing a mental disorder and receiving appropriate treatment and support. The longer the delay in getting help, the more difficult recovery can be.[27] It is important that people get support from family, friends, and work colleagues during this time. People are more likely to seek help if someone close to them suggests it.[28] **It is during this early intervention phase that mental health first aid can play an important role.**

Treatment and Supports

There are many different types of treatment and support. Once the person has made the decision to seek help, he or she may choose from a number of treatment approaches and service settings. There is no "one size fits all" approach. The range of people who can help persons with mental disorders includes primary care physicians, mental health professionals, psychiatrists, peer support specialists, and family and friends.

>> **Medical treatments** include various types of prescribed medications and other treatments given by a physician.

>> **Psychological treatments** involve providing a supportive relationship and changing the way the person thinks or behaves. Usually it is talking face to face with a mental health professional, or sometimes in a group, to address issues and to promote personal growth and coping skills.

>> **Complementary treatment and lifestyle changes** involve using natural or alternative therapies and changing the way one lives.

>> **Peer support groups** bring people with common problems together to share experiences and help each other. Participation in mutual aid self-help groups can help reduce feelings of isolation, increase knowledge, and enhance coping skills as well as bolster self-esteem. Family, friends, and faith community networks can be an important source of support for a person.

>> **Rehabilitation programs,** including the use of peer support specialists, help people regain skills and confidence to live and work more satisfactorily and successfully in their communities. Mental health first aid can continue to play an important role in this period if relapses or crises occur. At such times, people need support from those around them, particularly if no expert help is immediately available.

Recovery from Mental Disorders

Recovery is a personal journey with the goals of hope, empowerment, and autonomy. Too many Americans are unaware that mental disorders can be treated and recovery is possible.

In 2003, the final report of the President's New Freedom Commission on Mental Health, *Achieving the Promise: Transforming Mental Health Care in America*, called for recovery to be the "common, recognized outcome of mental health services," stating emphatically "the goal of mental health services is recovery."[4] In this report, *recovery* was defined as "the process in which people are able to live, work, learn, and participate fully in their communities. For some individuals, recovery is the ability to live a fulfilling and productive life despite a disability. For others, recovery implies the reduction or complete remission of symptoms."

Many factors contribute to recovery. These can include support of family and friends, availability of treatments, and getting early and appropriate treatment. It also includes opportunities for education and employment, support from others experiencing similar issues, and the ability and willingness of the person to participate in their own recovery.

Professionals Who Can Help

A variety of health professionals can provide help to a person with a mental disorder:

Primary Care Physician

For many who may be developing a mental disorder, their primary care physician may be the first professional they turn to for help. A primary care physician can recognize developing symptoms and provide the following types of help:

- Determining a possible physical cause

- Providing knowledge about the illness and suggestions for help

- Prescribing medication if needed

- Referring the person to a mental health professional

- Referring the person to a psychiatrist, particularly if the symptoms are severe or long lasting

- Linking the person to community support.

Mental Health Professionals

Licensed mental health professionals (such as clinical social workers, psychiatric nurse practitioners, psychologists, licensed counselors) specialize in the treatment of mental health problems. They are not medical doctors, but in some states, nurse practitioners and psychologists can prescribe some types of medications.

People who want help from a licensed mental health professional can contact one themselves (such as looking up a therapist in the Yellow

Pages), get a recommendation from their primary care physician, and ask friends or family members. Health insurance and managed care organizations have different levels of coverage for mental health services. For people without health insurance, help may be available from a community mental health center, federally qualified healthcare center, or other local health resources. Additionally, many religious organizations have counseling available. If you wish to have your services reimbursed by insurance, contact the insurance provider or primary care physician.

Certified Peer Specialists

Many who are on the road to recovery seek to share their experiences and help others by becoming a certified peer specialist. These specialists receive training that enables them to use their own experiences to promote hope, personal responsibility, empowerment, education, and self-determination.

Psychiatrists

Psychiatrists are medical doctors who specialize in the treatment of mental disorders. Psychiatrists focus on treating people with severe and/or long-lasting disorders. They are experts in medication and can help people suffering side effects or interactions with other medications. A primary care physician might refer a patient to a psychiatrist if the person is very ill or is not getting better quickly. Most psychiatrists work in private practice, at mental health centers, or in hospitals.

Transformation of Mental Health Care in the United States

The President's New Freedom Commission on Mental Health final report in 2003 recommended a fundamental transformation in the approach to mental health care in the United States.[4] This report recommended six goals to improve the lives of people with mental disorders:

GOAL 1	Americans understand that mental health is essential to overall health.
GOAL 2	Mental health care is consumer and family driven.
GOAL 3	Disparities in mental health services are eliminated.
GOAL 4	Early mental health screening, assessment, and referral to services are common practice.
GOAL 5	Excellent mental health care is delivered and research is accelerated.
GOAL 6	Technology is used to access mental health care and information.

Furthermore, the Commission developed the following vision statement:

> "We envision a future when everyone with a mental illness will recover, a future when mental illnesses can be prevented or cured, a future when mental illnesses are detected early, and a future when everyone with a mental illness at any stage of life has access to effective treatment and supports essentials for living, working, learning, and participating fully in the community."

Mental Health First Aid® is one piece of the jigsaw puzzle that will help to achieve these goals and assist in making the vision a reality.

Helpful Resources

WEBSITES

Mental Health America

www.mentalhealthamerica.net

Visit Mental Health America's site for information on mental health, getting help, and taking action.

National Council for Behavioral Health

www.TheNationalCouncil.org

To locate mental health and addictions treatment facilities in your community, use the Find a Provider feature on the National Council's website.

National Empowerment Center

www.power2u.org

The mission of the National Empowerment Center is to carry a message of recovery, empowerment, hope, and healing to those diagnosed with a mental illness. The center provides information and advocacy resources.

National Institute of Mental Health

PREVALENCE OF MENTAL DISORDERS IN AMERICA

www.nimh.nih.gov/health/publications/
the-numbers-count-mental-disorders-in-
america.shtml

The National Institute of Mental Health website provides statistics pertaining to mental disorders, including prevalence data by age, sex, race, and average age of onset.

President's New Freedom Commission on Mental Health

govinfo.library.unt.edu/mentalhealth
commission/reports/reports.htm

This commission report was released in 2003 as part of an effort to eliminate inequality for Americans with disabilities. It was tasked to "promote successful community integration for adults with a serious mental illness and children with a serious emotional disturbance." The final report describes problems and gaps in the U.S. mental health system and makes recommendations for improvements at the federal, state, and local levels of government, as well as private and public health care providers. A key recommendation calls for a "recovery-oriented mental health system."

World Health Organization

DISABILITY FROM MENTAL ILLNESS

www.who.int/topics/global_burden_of_
disease/en/

The World Health Organization web site contains information on the global burden of disease in various parts of the world, including burden due to mental disorders. It gives projections into future years, when the burden of mental disorders is expected to greatly increase.

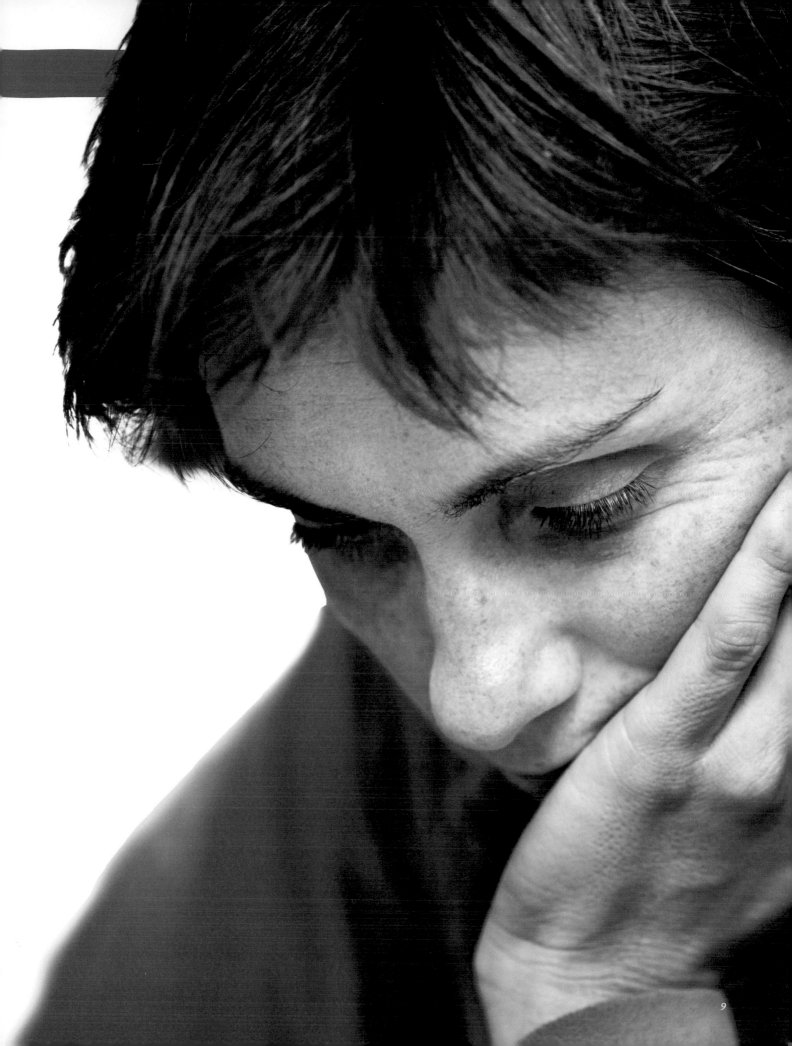

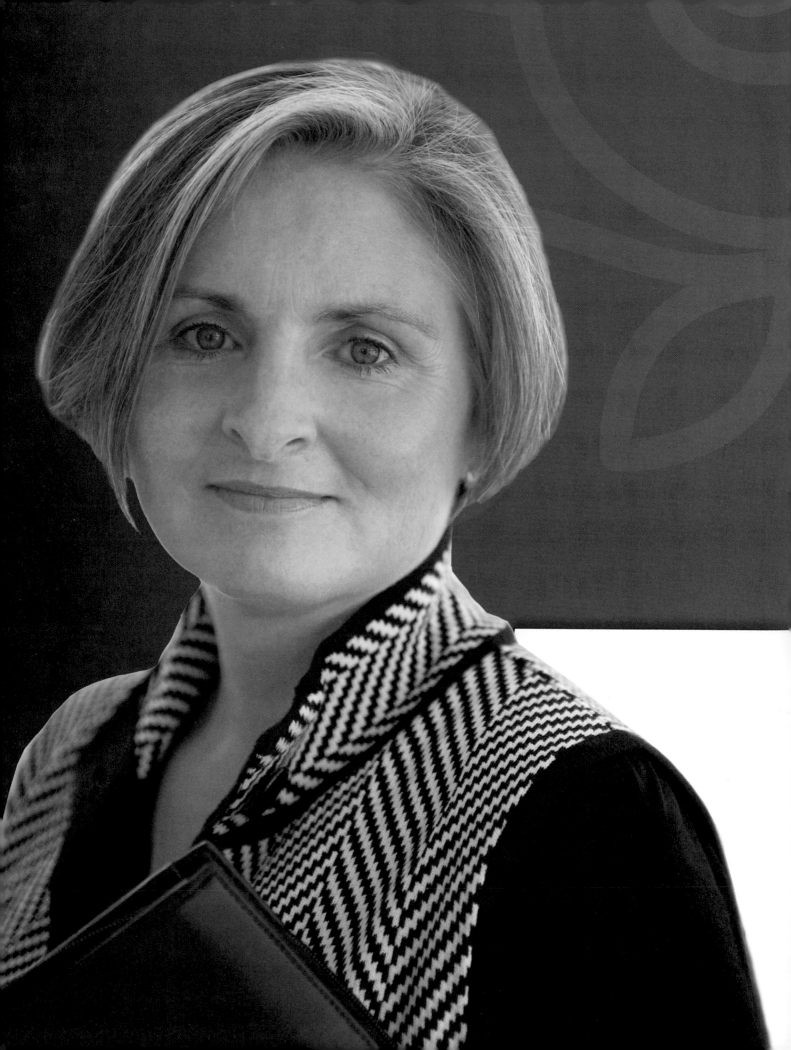

CHAPTER 2

Mental Health First Aid®

First aid is the help given to a person who is injured before professional medical treatment can be obtained. The aims of any first aid are to

1. Preserve life

2. Prevent further harm

3. Promote recovery

4. Provide comfort to the person who is ill or injured.

Mental Health First Aid is the help offered to a person developing a mental health problem or experiencing a mental health crisis. The first aid is given until appropriate treatment and support are received or until the crisis resolves.

The aims of Mental Health First Aid are to

1. Preserve life when a person may be a danger to self or others

2. Provide help to prevent the problem from becoming more serious

3. Promote and enhance recovery

4. Provide comfort and support.

Mental Health First Aid teaches the public how to recognize symptoms of mental health problems, how to offer and provide initial help, and how to guide a person toward appropriate treatments and other supportive help. Mental Health First Aid does not teach people to be therapists.

Why Mental Health First Aid?

There are many reasons why people can benefit from training in Mental Health First Aid:

>> **Mental health problems are common**, especially depression, anxiety, and misuse of alcohol and other drugs.[1] In the United States, more than half of adults (57.4 percent)[2] will experience a mental disorder during their lifetime. Every year, one in five (19.6 percent) is affected.[1] Throughout the course of a person's life, it is highly likely an individual will develop a mental health problem or have close contact with someone who does.

>> **Many people are not well informed** about how to recognize mental health problems, how to respond, or what effective treatments are available.[29] There are many myths and misunderstandings about mental health problems. Common myths include the idea that people with mental disorders are dangerous, that it is better to avoid psychiatric treatment, that people can use willpower to pull themselves out of mental health problems, and that only weak people have mental health problems. Lack of knowledge may result in denial and avoidance. With greater community knowledge about mental health problems, people will be able to recognize problems in others and better prepared to offer support.

>> **Many people with mental health problems do not seek help or delay seeking help.** In the United States, only 41 percent of the people who had a mental disorder in the past year received professional health care or other services.[30] Even when people seek treatment, many wait for years before doing so. For

example, half the people who seek help for depression delay seeking help for 8 years or more.[31] The longer the delay, the more difficult their recovery can be.[27] People with mental health problems are more likely to seek help if someone close to them suggests it.[28]

>> **There is stigma associated with mental health problems.** Stigma involves negative attitudes (prejudice) and negative behavior (discrimination). Stigma can lead people to hide their problems and delay seeking help.[31] People are often ashamed to discuss mental health problems with family, friends, teachers, and/or work colleagues and may be reluctant to seek treatment and support because of concerns about what others will think. Stigma can lead to exclusion of people with mental health problems from employment, housing, social activities, and relationships. People with mental health problems can internalize the stigma and begin to believe the negative things others say about them. Better understanding of the experiences of people with mental health problems can reduce stigma and discrimination.

>> **People with mental health problems may not have the insight that they need help or may be unaware that effective help is available.** Some mental health problems can cloud a person's thinking and rational decision-making processes, or the person can be in such severe distress that they cannot take effective action. In this situation, people close to them can facilitate appropriate help.

>> **Professional and other support services are not always available when a mental health problem arises.** There are professional people (primary care physicians, nurse practitioners, social workers, counselors, psychologists, and psychiatrists) and other support services that can help people with mental health problems. When these sources of help are not available, members of the public can offer immediate first aid and assist the person to get appropriate help and support.

The Mental Health First Aid Action Plan

In order to be able to give appropriate help, first aiders need basic knowledge about mental health problems to allow them to recognize that a disorder may be developing. It is important not to ignore symptoms or assume that they will just go away. It is also important not to lie or make excuses for the person's behavior, as this may delay getting assistance. The first aider needs to approach the person and see if there is anything they can do to assist him or her.

In any first aid course, participants learn an action plan to help someone who is injured or ill. The most common mnemonic, or memory device, used to remember the procedure is ABC, which stands for Airway, Breathing, and Circulation. Similarly, Mental Health First Aid provides an action plan on how to help a person in a mental health crisis. Its mnemonic is ALGEE® (see box).

MENTAL HEALTH FIRST AID ACTION PLAN	
ACTION A	Assess for risk of suicide or harm
ACTION L	Listen nonjudgmentally
ACTION G	Give reassurance and information
ACTION E	Encourage appropriate professional help *can start w/ primary care doctre*
ACTION E®	Encourage self-help and other support strategies

ACTION A: Assess for risk of suicide or harm

As in any first aid action plan, the initial task of assessment involves approaching the person to determine if there is a problem, assessing for any crises, and assisting the person in dealing with those crises. Possible crises might include the following:

- The person may harm himself or herself (by attempting suicide, using substances to become intoxicated, engaging in self-injury, or attempting to achieve extreme weight loss)

- The person experiences extreme distress (such as a panic attack or reaction to a traumatic event)

- The person's behavior is very disturbing to others (they become aggressive or lose touch with reality).

If the person appears to be at risk of harming self or others, the first aider must seek professional help immediately, even if the person does not want it.

Although the action of assisting with a crisis is the highest priority, other actions may need to occur first. These actions are not necessarily steps to be followed in a fixed order. The first aider needs to use good judgment about the order of these actions and be flexible and responsive to the person receiving help.

ACTION L: Listen nonjudgmentally

Listening to the person is very important. Most people experiencing distressing emotions and thoughts want an empathic listener first before being offered helpful options and resources. When listening nonjudgmentally, success comes when the first aider adopts certain attitudes and uses verbal and nonverbal listening skills that

- Allow the listener to really hear and understand what is being said

- Make it easier for the other person to feel they can talk freely without being judged.

ACTION G: Give reassurance and information

Once a person with a mental health problem feels that he or she has been heard, it becomes easier to offer encouragement and information. Reassurance includes emotional support, such as empathizing with how the person feels and voicing hope, as well as offering practical help with tasks that may seem overwhelming at the moment. Also, the first aider can offer to provide some information about mental health problems.

ACTION E: Encourage appropriate professional help

People with mental health problems will generally have a better recovery if they get appropriate professional help. However, they may not know about various options available to them. Such options include medication, counseling or psychological therapy, support for family members, assistance with vocational and educational goals, and assistance with income and accommodation.

ACTION E: Encourage self-help and other support strategies

Encourage the person to use self-help strategies or seek support of family, friends, and others. Peer supporters—others who have experienced mental health problems—can provide valuable help in the person's recovery.

IT IS IMPORTANT TO CARE FOR YOURSELF

After providing mental health first aid to a person in distress, you may feel worn out, frustrated, or even angry. You also may need to deal with the feelings and reactions you set aside during the encounter. It can be helpful to find someone to talk to about what has happened. If you do this, though, you need to remember to respect privacy; if you talk to someone, don't share the name of the person you helped or personal details that might identify him or her.

APPLYING THE MHFA ACTION PLAN TO DEVELOPING MENTAL HEALTH PROBLEMS AND CRISES

The second section in this manual explains how to apply the Mental Health First Aid Action Plan to the following developing mental health problems:

■ Depression

■ Anxiety disorders

■ Psychosis

■ Substance use disorders

■ Eating disorders.

The third section describes the best ways to assist a person experiencing a mental health crisis. The following are covered:

1. Suicidal thoughts and behaviors

2. Nonsuicidal self-injury

3. Panic attacks

4. Traumatic events affecting adults

5. Traumatic events affecting children

6. Acute psychosis

7. Medical emergency from alcohol abuse

8. Aggressive behavior

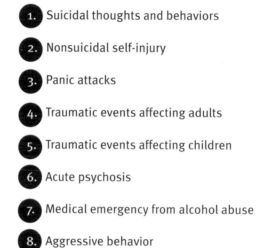

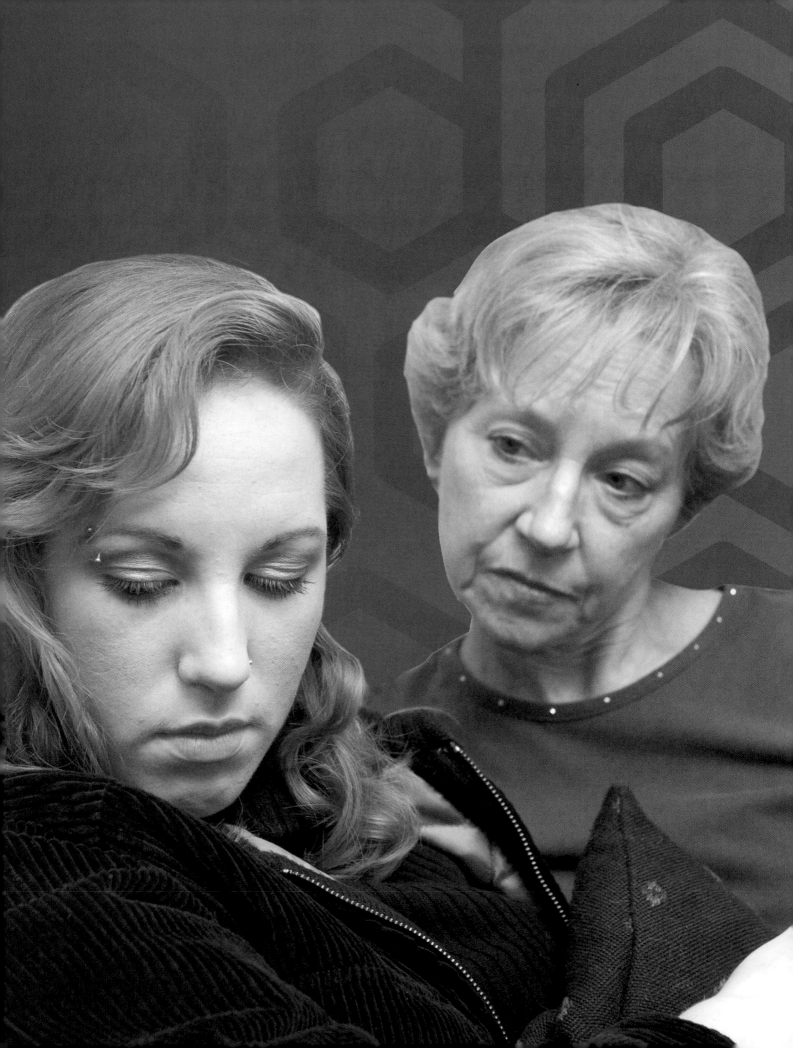

CHAPTER 3

Depression

What Is Depression?

The word *depression* is used in many different ways. People feel sad or blue when bad things happen. However, everyday "blues" or sadness is not a depressive disorder. We all may have a short-term depressed mood, but we cope and soon recover without treatment. A major depressive disorder lasts for at least two weeks and affects a person's ability to work, to carry out usual daily activities, and to have satisfying personal relationships.

Mood disorders affect nearly 1 of 10 U.S. adults in a given year.[1] The most common is major depressive disorder, which affects 6.8 percent of adults in any one year. The median age of onset is 32 years,[2] meaning that half the people who will ever have an episode will have had their first episode by this age. Depression often co-occurs with anxiety or substance use disorders. Depression is more common in females than in males. It often recurs. Once a person has had an occurrence of depression, they are prone to subsequent episodes.[32]

Symptoms of Depression[21]

A person who is clinically depressed would have at least one of these two symptoms, nearly every day, for at least 2 weeks:

■ An unusually sad mood

■ Loss of enjoyment and interest in activities that used to be enjoyable

The person also might have these symptoms:

■ Lack of energy and tiredness

■ Feeling worthless or feeling guilty though not really at fault

■ Thinking often about death or wishing to be dead

■ Difficulty concentrating or making decisions

■ Moving more slowly or sometimes becoming agitated and unable to settle

■ Having sleeping difficulties or sometimes sleeping too much

■ Loss of interest in food or sometimes eating too much. Changes in eating habits may lead to either loss of weight or weight gain.

Not every person who is depressed has all these symptoms. People differ in the number and severity of symptoms. Even if the symptoms don't add up to an official diagnosis of a depressive disorder, the impact on life can still be significant.

Symptoms of depression affect emotions, thinking, behavior, and physical well-being. Some examples are as follows:

›› EMOTIONS

Sadness, anxiety, guilt, anger, mood swings, lack of emotional responsiveness, feelings of helplessness, hopelessness, irritability.

>> THOUGHTS

Frequent self-criticism, self-blame, worry, pessimism, impaired memory and concentration, indecisiveness and confusion, a tendency to believe others see you in a negative light, thoughts of death and suicide.

>> BEHAVIOR

Crying spells, withdrawal from others, neglect of responsibilities, loss of interest in personal appearance, loss of motivation, slowed down, using alcohol or other drugs.

>> PHYSICAL

Chronic fatigue, lack of energy, sleeping too much or too little, overeating or loss of appetite, constipation, weight loss or gain, headaches, irregular menstrual cycle, loss of sexual desire, unexplained aches and pains.

How a Person with Depression May Appear

A person who is depressed may be slow in moving and thinking, although agitation can occur. Even speech can be slow and monotonous. There can be a lack of interest and attention to personal hygiene and grooming. The person usually looks sad and depressed and is often anxious, irritable, and easily moved to tears. Mild depression may be successfully hidden from others, while with severe depression, the person may be emotionally unresponsive and described as "beyond tears."

The thinking of a person with clinical depression often has themes of hopelessness and helplessness, with a negative self-image: *I'm a failure. It's all my fault. Nothing good ever happens to me. I'm worthless. No one loves me.* Or there may be pessimism about life or the future: *Life is not worth living. There is nothing good out there. Things will always be bad.*

Other Mood Disorders

Bipolar Disorder

People with bipolar disorder (previously called *manic depressive disorder*) have extreme mood swings. They can experience periods of depression, periods of mania, and long periods of normal mood in between. The time between these different episodes varies greatly from person to person. Approximately 2.8 percent of U.S. adults experience bipolar disorder in any given year.[1] The median age of onset is 25 years, which means that half the people with bipolar disorder will have had their first episode by this age.[2] Bipolar disorder is equally common in males and females.

Depression experienced by a person with bipolar disorder has some or all of the symptoms of depression listed previously. A person cannot be diagnosed with bipolar disorder until he or she has experienced both an episode of mania and an episode of depression. It may, therefore, take many years before an accurate diagnosis is made and appropriate treatment provided.

Mania appears to be the opposite of depression. A person experiencing mania will have an elevated mood, be overconfident, and be full of energy. The person might be very talkative and full of ideas, have less need for sleep, and take uncharacteristic risks. Although some of these symptoms may sound beneficial, such as increased energy and being full of ideas, they often get people into difficult situations. They could spend too much money and get into debt, become angry and aggressive, get into legal trouble, or be sexually promiscuous. These consequences may cause havoc with work, study, and personal relationships. The person can have grandiose ideas and may lose touch with reality (that is, become psychotic). In fact, it is not unusual for people with this disorder to become psychotic during depressive or manic episodes.[33, 34] Additional information on bipolar disorder is discussed in Chapter 5.

Depression Following Childbirth

A recent national survey of U.S. women found a 50 percent higher risk of developing a major depressive disorder[35] in the 12-month period following childbirth. Contributing factors are hormonal and physical changes and the responsibilities of caring for the baby. Feeling sad or having the "baby blues" after giving birth is common, but when these feelings last for more than two weeks, this may be a sign of a depressive disorder. Having had a previous episode of depression increases risk for postpartum depression, and symptoms often already are present during pregnancy.

Depressive disorder following childbirth is called *postpartum* or *postnatal depression*. The symptoms do not differ from depression at other times. However, depression at this time has an impact not only on the mother, but also on the mother–infant relationship and on the child's cognitive and emotional development. For this reason, it is particularly important to get good treatment for postpartum depression. Treatment not only helps the mother's depressive symptoms, but also can improve the mother–child relationship and the child's cognitive development.[36]

Seasonal Depression

Seasonal affective disorder (SAD) is characterized by a depressive illness during the fall and winter months, when there is less natural sunlight. Prevalence increases with higher latitudes. The depression generally lifts during spring and summer. People with SAD are more likely to experience the following symptoms of depression: lack of energy, sleeping too much, overeating, weight gain, and a craving for carbohydrates.[21]

What Causes Depression?

Depression has no single cause and often involves the interaction of many diverse biological, psychological, and social factors. People may become depressed when something very distressing has happened and they feel powerless to control the situation, such as the following:

■ A breakup of a relationship or living in conflict

■ Long-term poverty

■ Loss of a job or difficulty finding a new one

■ Having an accident that results in long-term disability

■ Bullying or victimization

■ Being a victim of crime

■ Developing a long-term physical illness

■ Death of a partner, family member, or friend

Depression also can result from

■ The effects of medical conditions; for example, Parkinson's disease, Huntington's disease, stroke, vitamin B12 deficiency, hypothyroidism, systemic lupus erythematosus, hepatitis, mononucleosis, HIV, some cancers [21]

■ Having a baby (see Depression Following Childbirth)

■ The side effects of certain medications or drugs

■ The stress of having another mental disorder, such as schizophrenia, an anxiety disorder, or an eating disorder

- Intoxication or withdrawal from alcohol or other drugs

- Premenstrual changes in hormone levels

- Lack of exposure to bright light in the winter months *(see Seasonal Depression)*

- Caring full-time for a person with a long-term disability.

Some people will develop depression in a distressing situation, whereas others in the same situation may not. Those most prone to develop depression are

- People who previously have had an episode of depression

- People who have family members who have had episodes of depression

- People with a more sensitive emotional nature

- People who have had a difficult childhood (for example, those who experienced physical, sexual, or emotional abuse, neglect, or overstrictness)

- Females.

Depression is believed to be caused by changes in natural brain chemicals called neurotransmitters. These chemicals send messages from one nerve cell to another. When a person becomes depressed, the brain has fewer of these chemical messengers. One of these is serotonin, a mood-regulating brain chemical. Many antidepressant medications work by changing the activity of serotonin in the brain.

Importance of Early Intervention for Depression

Early intervention is important. People who have one episode of depression are prone to subsequent episodes. They fall into depression more easily with each subsequent episode.[32] For this reason, some people go on to have repeated episodes throughout life. To prevent this pattern from occurring, it is important to intervene early with a first episode of depression to make sure it is treated quickly and effectively.

The Mental Health First Aid Action Plan for Depression[37]

MENTAL HEALTH FIRST AID ACTION PLAN	
ACTION A	Assess for risk of suicide or harm
ACTION L	Listen nonjudgmentally
ACTION G	Give reassurance and information
ACTION E	Encourage appropriate professional help
ACTION E®	Encourage self-help and other support strategies

ACTION A: Assess for risk of suicide or harm[38]

If you think someone you know may be depressed and in need of help, approach the person about your concerns. It is important to choose a suitable time when you and the person are available to talk, as well as a space where you both feel comfortable. Let the person know that you are available to talk

when they are ready; do not pressure the person to talk right away. It can be helpful to let the person choose the moment to open up. However, if the person does not initiate a conversation, you can begin a dialogue. Respect the person's privacy and confidentiality unless you are concerned the person is at risk of harming self or others.

The main crises associated with depression are as follows:

- The person has *suicidal thoughts and behaviors*.

- The person is engaging in *nonsuicidal self-injury*.

If you have no concerns that the person is in crisis, you may ask them how they are feeling and how long they have been feeling that way, and then move on to Action L.

FACTS ON SUICIDE IN THE UNITED STATES

>> A national survey of U.S. adults found that in a 12-month period, 2.6 percent thought about suicide, 0.7 percent made a plan, and 0.4 percent attempted suicide.[39]

>> Suicide is the 11th most common cause of death.[40] In 2005, suicide took the lives of 32,637 people (.011 percent of the population). They left behind friends, families, and whole communities scarred by this loss.

>> Suicide is the second leading cause of death among 25 to 34 year-olds and the third leading cause of death among 15-to 24-year-olds.[41]

>> In 2007, 14.5 percent of U.S. high school students reported that they had seriously considered attempting suicide during the 12 months preceding the survey. More than 6.9 percent of students reported they had actually attempted suicide one or more times during the same period.[42]

>> Males take their own lives at nearly four times the rate of females, but women attempt suicide about two to three times as often as men.[40]

>> Among males, adults 75 and older have the highest rate of suicide. Among females, those in their 40s and 50s have the highest rate of suicide.[40]

>> Alcohol or other drugs were found in more than one third of completed suicide toxicology reports done in 13 states in 2005.[43]

>> Approximately 87 percent of people who complete suicide have a mental disorder.[44]

Having depression increases the risk of suicide. Of the people who complete suicide, 43 percent had a mood disorder.[44] A person may feel so overwhelmed and helpless about life events that the future appears hopeless. The person may think suicide is the only way out. However, not every person who is depressed is at risk for suicide, nor is everyone who is at risk for suicide necessarily depressed. Encourage people to talk about their feelings, symptoms, and what is going on in their mind. Be alert for any of the warning signs of suicide (see the following box).

Warning Signs of Suicide[45]

■ Threatening to hurt or kill himself or herself

■ Looking for ways to kill himself or herself, seeking access to pills, weapons, or other means

■ Talking or writing about death, dying, or suicide

■ Expressing hopelessness

■ Feeling rage or anger, seeking revenge

■ Acting recklessly or engaging in risky activities, seemingly without thinking

■ Feeling trapped, like there is no way out

■ Increasing alcohol or drug use

■ Withdrawing from friends, family, or society

■ Experiencing anxiety or agitation, being unable to sleep, or sleeping all the time

■ Undergoing dramatic changes in mood

■ Feeling no reason for living, no sense of purpose in life

People may show one or many of these signs, and some may show signs not listed.

If you have seen warning signs, engage the person in a discussion about your observations. If you suspect someone may be at risk of suicide, it is important to directly ask about suicidal thoughts. Do not avoid using the word *suicide*. It is important to ask the question without dread and without expressing a negative judgment. The question must be direct and to the point. For example, you could ask,

■ "Are you having thoughts of suicide?"

■ "Are you thinking about killing yourself?"

If you appear confident in the face of a suicide crisis, this can be reassuring for the suicidal person. Although some people think that asking about suicide can put the idea in the person's mind, *this is not true.* Another myth is that someone who talks about suicide isn't really serious. Remember that talking about suicide may be a way for the person to indicate just how badly they feel.

FACTS ON NONSUICIDAL SELF-INJURY

Many terms are used to describe self-injury, including *self-harm, self-mutilation, cutting,* and *parasuicide.* There is a great deal of debate about what self-injury is and how it is different from suicidal behavior. Here, the term *nonsuicidal self-injury* is used to refer to situations where self-injury has no suicidal intent. It is not easy to tell the difference between nonsuicidal self-injury and a suicide attempt. The only way to know is to ask the person directly, "Are you suicidal?"

There are many different types of nonsuicidal self-injury, including [46]

■ Cutting, scratching, or pinching skin enough to cause bleeding or a mark that remains on the skin

■ Banging or punching objects to the point of bruising or bleeding

■ Ripping and tearing skin

■ Carving words or patterns into skin

■ Interfering with the healing of wounds

■ Burning skin with cigarettes, matches, or hot water

■ Pulling out large amounts of hair

■ Deliberately overdosing on medications when this is *not* meant as a suicide attempt.

Nonsuicidal self-injury is common in young people. A survey of U.S. college students found that 17 percent had engaged in nonsuicidal self-injury at some time in their lives.[46] Another survey of high school students

found that 20 percent of girls and 9 percent of boys had engaged in nonsuicidal self-injury. These young people reported more emotional distress, more anger problems, lower self-esteem, more risky health behaviors, and more antisocial behaviors.[47]

People who engage in nonsuicidal self-injury do so for many reasons, including [48]

- To escape unbearable anguish

- To change the behavior of others

- To escape from a situation

- To show desperation to others

- To get back at other people or make them feel guilty

- To relieve tension

- To seek help.

Recent research suggests that adolescents may be more likely to engage in nonsuicidal self-injury when close friends or other peers engage in similar behaviors.[49]

Let the person know that you are concerned and are willing to help.

- If there is concern about **suicidal thoughts**, see *First Aid for Suicidal Thoughts and Behaviors*.

  If you have serious concerns, call 911 or the National Suicide Prevention Lifeline at 1-800-273-TALK (8255).

- If there is concern about **nonsuicidal self-injury**, see *First Aid for Nonsuicidal Self-Injury*.

ACTION L: Listen nonjudgmentally

If you believe the person is *not in a crisis* that needs immediate attention, you can engage the person in conversation, such as asking how they are feeling and how long they have been feeling this way. Listening nonjudgmentally is important at this stage as it can help the person to feel heard and understood while not being judged in any way. This can make it easy for the person to feel comfortable and talk freely about their problems or ask for help.

TIPS FOR NONJUDGMENTAL LISTENING

It is tough to be nonjudgmental all of the time. We automatically make judgments about people from the minute we first see or meet them based on appearance, behavior, and what they say. Nonjudgmental listening is not about avoiding those judgments—it is about ensuring that you don't express those negative judgments, as this can get in the way of helping. If you have decided to approach someone with your concerns, it is a good idea to spend some time reflecting on your own state of mind first to ensure you are in the right frame of mind to talk and listen without being judgmental.

Although the focus of your conversation is the person's feelings, thoughts, and experiences, you need to be aware of your own. Helping someone in distress may evoke an unexpected emotional response in you; you may find yourself feeling fearful, overwhelmed, sad, or even irritated or frustrated.

In spite of any emotional response you have, you need to continue listening respectfully and avoid expressing any negative reaction. This is sometimes difficult and may be made more complex by your relationship with the person or your personal beliefs about the situation. You need to set aside these beliefs and reactions in order to focus on the needs of the person you are helping to be heard, understood, and helped. Remember, you are providing people with a safe space to express themselves, and a negative reaction may block that sense of safety.

Effective Communication Skills for Nonjudgmental Listening

You can be an effective nonjudgmental listener by paying special attention to two areas:

■ Your *attitudes*, and how they are conveyed, and

■ Effective *communication skills*, both verbal and nonverbal.

ATTITUDES
The key attitudes are acceptance, genuineness, and empathy.

›› Adopting an attitude of *acceptance* means respecting the person's feelings, personal values, and experiences as valid, even if they are different from your own or you disagree with them. Do not judge, criticize, or trivialize what the person says because of your own beliefs or attitudes. This may mean withholding any and all judgments that you have made about the person and his or her circumstances.

›› *Genuineness* means that what you say and do shows that you are accepting of the person. This means not holding one set of attitudes while expressing another. Your body language and verbal cues should reinforce your acceptance of the person. For example, if you tell the person you accept and respect their feelings, but maintain a defensive posture or avoid eye contact, the person will know you are not being genuine.

›› *Empathy* means being able to imagine yourself in the other person's place, showing them that they are truly heard and understood by you. This doesn't mean saying something glib such as "I understand exactly how you are feeling"—it is more appropriate to say that you can imagine what they might be going through. Remember that empathy is different from sympathy, which means feeling sorry for or pitying the person.

VERBAL SKILLS
Using the following simple verbal skills will show you are listening:

■ Ask questions that show you genuinely care, and seek clarification about what you are hearing.

■ Check your understanding by restating what they have said and summarizing facts and feelings.

■ Listen not only to what the person says, but how it is said; tone of voice and nonverbal cues will give extra clues about feelings.

■ Use minimal prompts, such as "I see" and "ah," when necessary to keep the conversation going.

■ Be patient, even when the person may not be communicating well, is repetitive, or is speaking more slowly and less clearly than usual.

■ Don't be critical, and don't express your frustration at the person for having such symptoms.

■ Avoid giving unhelpful advice such as "pull yourself together" or "cheer up."

■ Do not interrupt the person, especially to share your opinions or experiences.

■ Avoid confrontation unless necessary to prevent harmful or dangerous acts.

Remember that pauses and silences are okay. Silence can be uncomfortable for many people, but the person may need time to think about what has been said or may be struggling to find the right words. Interrupting the silence may make it difficult for them to get back on track and may damage the rapport you have been building. Consider whether the silence is awkward, or just awkward for you.

NONVERBAL SKILLS

Nonverbal communications and body language express a great deal. Good nonverbal skills show you are listening, while poor nonverbal skills can damage the rapport and negate what you say.

Keep the following nonverbal cues in mind:

- Pay close attention to what the person says.

- Maintain comfortable eye contact. Don't avoid eye contact, but do avoid staring; you can do this by maintaining a level of eye contact that seems most comfortable to the person.

- Maintain an open body position. Don't cross your arms over your body, as this may appear defensive.

- Sit down, even if the person is standing, as this seems less threatening.

- It is best to sit alongside and angled toward the person rather than directly opposite him or her.

- Do not fidget.

CULTURAL CONSIDERATIONS FOR NONJUDGMENTAL LISTENING

If you are assisting someone from a cultural background different from your own, you may need to adjust some verbal and nonverbal behaviors. For example, the person may be comfortable with a level of eye contact different from what you are used to or may be used to more personal space.

If these differences are interfering with your ability to be an effective helper, it may be helpful to explore and try to understand the person's experiences, values, or belief systems. Be prepared to discuss what is culturally appropriate and realistic for the person, or seek advice from someone from the same cultural background before engaging him or her.

ACTION G: Give reassurance and information

TREAT THE PERSON WITH RESPECT AND DIGNITY

Each person's situation and needs are unique. It is important to respect the person's autonomy while considering the extent to which the person is able to make personal decisions. Respect the person's privacy and confidentiality unless you are concerned that the person is at risk of harming self or others.

DO NOT BLAME THE PERSON FOR THE ILLNESS

Depression is a real health problem. It is important to remind the person that it is a health problem and they are not to blame for feeling "down."

HAVE REALISTIC EXPECTATIONS

Accept the person as he or she is, and have realistic expectations. Everyday activities like cleaning house, paying bills, or feeding the dog may seem overwhelming. Let the person know that personal weakness or failure is not the cause of depression and that you don't think less of them as a person. Acknowledge that the person is not "faking," "lazy," "weak," or "selfish."

OFFER CONSISTENT EMOTIONAL SUPPORT AND UNDERSTANDING

It is more important for you to be genuinely caring than for you to say all the right things. The person really needs additional love and understanding to get through the illness, so be empathic, compassionate, and patient. People with depression are often overwhelmed by irrational fears; you need to gently understand. It is important to be patient, persistent, and encouraging when supporting someone with depression. Offer the person kindness and attention, even if it is not reciprocated. Let the person know that there is no risk of abandonment. Be consistent and predictable in your interactions with the person.

GIVE THE PERSON HOPE FOR RECOVERY

Reassure the person that, with time and treatment, they will feel better. Offer emotional support and hope for a more positive future in whatever acceptable form they will accept.

PROVIDE PRACTICAL HELP

Offer the person practical assistance with tasks, but be careful not to take over or encourage dependency.

OFFER INFORMATION

Offer the person information about depression. If the response is positive, it is important that you give resources that are accurate and appropriate to the situation. Don't assume the person knows nothing about depression, because they, or someone else close to them, may have previously experienced depression.

What Isn't Supportive?

- Don't tell someone with depression to get better, as they cannot "snap out of it" or "get over it."

- Do not be hostile or sarcastic when the person attempts to be responsive, but rather accept these responses as the best the person has to offer at that time.

- Do not adopt an overinvolved or overprotective attitude toward someone who is depressed.

- Do not nag the person to try to get them to do what they normally would.

- Do not trivialize the person's experiences by pressuring them to "put a smile on your face," to "get your act together," or to "lighten up."

- Do not belittle or dismiss the person's feelings by attempting to say something positive like, "You don't seem that bad to me."

- Avoid speaking to the person in a patronizing tone of voice, and do not use overly compassionate looks of concern.

- Resist the urge to try to cure the person's depression or provide answers to their problems.
  Collaborate or get them connected to professional

ACTION E: Encourage appropriate professional help

Everybody feels down or sad at times, but it is important to be able to recognize when depression has become more than a temporary experience and when to encourage that person to seek professional help. Professional help is warranted when depression lasts for weeks and affects a person's functioning in daily life. Many with depressive disorders do not seek professional help. In the United States, only 57 percent of people who had major depressive disorder

in the past year received professional mental health care or other service.[30] Even when people do seek help, they can delay for many years.[31] These delays affect long-term recovery. People with depressive disorders are more likely to seek help if someone close to them suggests it.[28]

DISCUSS OPTIONS FOR SEEKING PROFESSIONAL HELP

Offer the person help to manage feelings. If they feel they do need help, discuss the options they have and encourage them to use these options. If the person does not know where to get help, offer to help them seek assistance. It is important to encourage the person to get appropriate professional help and effective treatment as early as possible. If the person would like you to support them by accompanying them to an appointment with a health professional, don't take over completely; a person with depression needs to make their own decisions as much as possible. Health professionals often do not recognize depression; it may take some time to get a diagnosis and find a healthcare provider with whom the person is able to establish a good relationship. Encourage the person not to give up seeking appropriate professional help.

PROFESSIONALS WHO CAN HELP

A variety of health professionals can provide help to a person with depression:

- Primary care physicians

- Mental health professionals

- Certified peer specialists

- Psychiatrists.

More information about these professionals can be found in Chapter 1.

Only in severe cases, or where there is a danger a person might harm himself or herself, is a depressed person admitted to a hospital. Most people with depression can be treated effectively in the community.

Treatments Available for Depression

Most people recover from depression and lead satisfying and productive lives. There is a range of effective treatments for depression.[50]

SUPPORTIVE COUNSELING

Supportive counseling involves being a good listener and providing emotional support. The therapist also may give information about depression and teach problem-solving skills. This type of treatment is most appropriate for mild depression.

PSYCHOLOGICAL THERAPIES

There is good evidence for psychological therapies that have been developed to treat depression, such as cognitive behavioral therapy (CBT) and interpersonal psychotherapy. CBT is based on the idea that how we think affects the way we feel. When people get depressed, they think negatively about most things. There may be thoughts about how hopeless the person's situation is and how helpless the person feels, with a negative view of himself or herself, the world, and the future. CBT helps the person recognize unhelpful thoughts and change them to more realistic ones. It also helps people change depressive behaviors by scheduling regular activities and engaging in pleasurable activities. It can include components such as stress management, relaxation techniques, and sleep management. Interpersonal psychotherapy helps people resolve conflict with others, deal with grief or changes in relationships, and develop better relationships. Research shows a better outcome when psychological therapy is given in combination with antidepressant medication. There is some evidence that a form of CBT, called dialectical behavior therapy, can be helpful for people who self-injure.[51] Its main goals are to teach coping skills for stress, to regulate emotions, and to improve relationships.

MEDICAL TREATMENT

Antidepressant medications have proven effective with adults who have depression. While controversial in the mental health community, electroconvulsive therapy (ECT) has been reported as effective for some adults with severe depression. However, ECT also has been known to cause negative side effects, such as memory loss. For people with bipolar disorder, mood stabilizer medications can help reduce the swings from one mood to another.

WHAT IF THE PERSON DOESN'T WANT HELP?

The person may not want to seek professional help. Find out if there are specific reasons why this is the case. For example, the person might be concerned about finances, not having a doctor they like, or being hospitalized. These reasons may be based on mistaken beliefs, or you may be able to help the person overcome worry about seeking help. If the person still doesn't want help after you have explored the reasons, let them know that if they change their mind about seeking help, they can contact you. Respect the person's right not to seek help unless you believe that they are at risk of harming self or others.

ACTION E: Encourage self-help and other support strategies

OTHER PEOPLE WHO CAN HELP

Encourage the person to consider other available support, such as family, friends, faith communities, support groups, or others who have experienced depression (peer supporters). Some people who experience depression find it helpful to meet with others who have had similar experiences. There is some evidence that these mutual help groups can help with recovery from depression and anxiety.[14] Family, friends, and faith community networks also can be an important source of support for a person who is depressed. Recovery from symptoms is quicker for people who feel supported by those around them.[52]

People with mental disorders who are hospitalized are less likely to receive flowers, get-well cards, or other gifts. This can lead to feelings of rejection. It is important that family and friends provide the same sort of support to an ill person with a mental disorder as they would to a person with a physical disorder.[53]

SELF-HELP STRATEGIES

People who are depressed frequently use self-help strategies. The person's ability and desire to use self-help strategies will depend on their interests and the severity of their depression. Therefore, do not be overly forceful when trying to encourage the person to use self-help strategies.

Lifestyle and complementary therapies that have some scientific evidence for effectiveness include[54]

>> **Exercise,** including aerobic (jogging or brisk walking) and anaerobic (weight training)

>> **SAMe** (S-Adenosyl methionine)—a compound made in the body and available as a supplement in drug stores

>> **St. John's wort** (hypericum perforatum)—an herbal remedy widely available in drug stores

>> **Self-help books** based on cognitive behavioral therapy (CBT; see Resources at end of chapter)

>> **Computerized therapy**—self-help treatment programs delivered over the Internet or on a computer; some are available free of charge (see Resources at end of chapter)

>> **Relaxation training** involves teaching a person to relax voluntarily by tensing and relaxing muscle groups; some programs are available from the Internet for free download (see Resources at end of chapter)

>> **Light therapy**—bright light exposure to the eyes, often in the morning.

In addition to seeking out scientific evidence of what treatments and supports work for depression, it is important to look at what consumers find helpful. A large Internet survey asked those who had received treatment for depression to rate the effectiveness of treatment. Rated as most effective were some antidepressant medications, CBT, interpersonal psychotherapy, other types of psychotherapy, and exercise.[55]

Helpful Resources

FOR DEPRESSION AND SUICIDAL INTENTIONS

WEBSITES

American Association of Suicidology

www.suicidology.org

Founded in 1968, the American Association of Suicidology (AAS) promotes research, public awareness programs, public education, and training for professionals and volunteers. In addition, AAS serves as a national clearinghouse for information on suicide.

American Foundation for Suicide Prevention

www.afsp.org

The American Foundation for Suicide Prevention (AFSP) provides information about suicide, support for survivors, prevention, research, and more. The Suicide Prevention Action Network merged with AFSP in 2009.

Brain & Behavior Research Foundation

bbrfoundation.org/

This site provides information and downloadable fact sheets on depressive disorders.

Mental Health America

www.mentalhealthamerica.net

Visit Mental Health America's site for information on mental health, getting help, and taking action.

DEPRESSION SCREENING

www.depression-screening.org

This website is sponsored by Mental Health America as part of the Campaign for America's Mental Health. The mission of this website is to educate people about clinical depression, offer a confidential way for people to get screened for symptoms of the illness, and guide people toward appropriate professional help if necessary.

MoodGYM

moodgym.anu.edu.au

This CBT website has been evaluated in a scientific trial and found to be effective in relieving depression symptoms if people work through it systematically.[56] This site teaches people to use ways of thinking that will help prevent depression.

National Alliance on Mental Illness

www.nami.org

NAMI is a nonprofit, grassroots, self-help, support and advocacy organization of individuals with mental disorders and their families. This website provides many resources on mental disorders, including depression, that are helpful for people who have experienced a mental illness and their families, including support groups, education, and training.

National Council for Behavioral Health

www.TheNationalCouncil.org

To locate mental health and addictions treatment facilities in your community, use the Find a Provider feature on the National Council's website.

National Institute of Mental Health

www.nimh.nih.gov

This U.S. government site gives a wealth of up-to-date information on depression and suicide in the form of downloadable booklets and fact sheets.

Postpartum Support International

www.postpartum.net

Postpartum Support International's (PSI's) website receives more than 100,000 visitors a year who resource PSI for support, education, and local providers. PSI's toll-free help line serves more than 1,000 callers a month and is staffed by a volunteer team of PSI-trained responders who rapidly refer callers to appropriate local resources, including emergency services. 800-944-4PPD (4773)

Progressive Relaxation

www.hws.edu/studentlife/counseling_relax.aspx

Two progressive relaxation tapes can be downloaded from the website of Hobart and William Smith Colleges in Geneva, New York.

Suicide Prevention Resource Center

www.sprc.org

The Suicide Prevention Resource Center has fact sheets on suicide by state and by population characteristics, as well as on many other subjects.

BOOKS

These two self-help books based on CBT for depression have been found effective in trials:

Burns, D. D. (1999) *Feeling good: the new mood therapy (revised edition)*. Quill Publishers, New York, NY.

Lewinsohn, P. M., Munoz, R. A., Youngren, M. A., Zeiss, A. M. (1992) *Control your depression (revised edition)*. Simon & Schuster, New York, NY.

Other books that may be useful:

Bieling, P. J. and Antony, M. M. (2003) *Ending the depression cycle*. New Harbinger Publications, Oakland, CA.
This is a depression relapse prevention workbook based on CBT principles.

Ellis, T. E. (1996) *Choosing to live: how to defeat suicide through cognitive therapy*. New Harbinger Publications, Oakland, CA.
This CBT-based self-help book focuses on learning thinking strategies for overcoming suicidal thoughts.

Greenburger, D., and Padesky, C. (1995) *Mind over mood: change how you feel by changing how you think*. Guilford Press, New York, NY.
This is a CBT-based self-help book for depression, anxiety, and interpersonal problems.

Knaus, W. J. (2012) *The cognitive behavioral workbook for depression, second edition: a step-by-step program*. New Harbinger Publications, Oakland, CA.
This CBT manual can be used alone or in conjunction with therapy. It also can be purchased as an eBook directly from the publisher (www.newharbinger.com).

HELP LINES

American Psychiatric Association Answer Center
1-888-35-PSYCH (77924)
Live operators available 8:30 a.m. to 6 p.m., Eastern time, refer you to local board-certified psychiatrists.

American Psychological Association Public Education Line
1-800-964-2000
Follow the automated instructions and press the number 1. Then an operator refers you to local board-certified psychologists.

National Suicide Prevention Lifeline
1-800-273-TALK (8255)
This hotline is available 24 hours a day. Phone calls are transferred to trained counselors in more than 130 sites nationwide. **This service has a new feature for veterans.** When veterans, their families, or friends call this number and press 1, they can talk to a trained, caring professional in a specialized veterans call center. Calls are free and confidential, 24 hours a day, 7 days a week. This feature of the hotline is a partnership between the Department of Veterans Affairs and the Substance Abuse and Mental Health Services Administration in the Department of Health and Human Services.

The Trevor Project
1-866-488-7386
www.thetrevorhelpline.org
This is a free and confidential suicide prevention help line for gay and questioning youth that offers hope and someone to talk to 24 hours a day.

SUPPORT GROUPS

American Self-Help Group Clearinghouse
www.mentalhelp.net/selfhelp/
A keyword-searchable database of 1,100 national, international, model, and online self-help support groups, including many for depression. Also listed are self-help clearinghouses worldwide, research studies, information on starting face-to-face and online groups, and a registry for persons interested in starting national or international self-help groups.

Depression and Bipolar Support Alliance
www.dbsalliance.org
On the home page of this website, click on "Find Support." You will be able to find out if a support group is meeting in your area. These are peer-led support groups.

National Alliance on Mental Illness
www.nami.org
NAMI is a nonprofit, grassroots, self-help, support and advocacy organization of individuals with mental disorders and their families. This website provides many resources on mental disorders, including depression, that are helpful for people who have experienced a mental illness and their families, including support groups, education, and training. On the home page, click on "Find Support."

Recovery International

www.lowselfhelpsystems.org/

On the home page, click on "Find a Meeting" to find the next Recovery International meeting in your area.

Recovery International, a Chicago-based self-help mental health organization, sponsors weekly group peer-led meetings in many communities, as well as telephone and Internet-based meetings.

Helpful Resources

FOR NONSUICIDAL SELF-INJURY

WEBSITES

Focus Adolescent Services

www.focusas.com

This website is designed for parents and covers a wide range of mental health problems; it has a section on self-injury. Information and resources can be obtained weekdays only, 9 a.m. to 5 p.m. Eastern time, at 410-341-4216.

S.A.F.E. Alternatives (Self-Abuse Finally Ends)

www.selfinjury.com

S.A.F.E. Alternatives is a residential treatment program for people who engage in self-injury. The website includes information about self-injury and information about starting treatment.

S.A.F.E. information line: 1-800-DON'T CUT (366-8288)

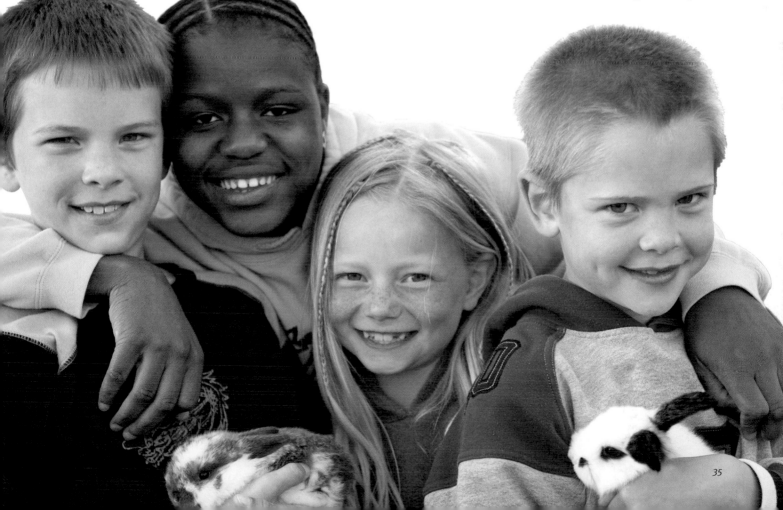

BOOKS

Conterio, K. and Lader, W. (1999) *Bodily harm: the breakthrough healing program for self-injurers.* Hyperion, New York, NY.
Written by the directors of the S.A.F.E. Alternatives program, this book is suitable for people who engage in self-injury and their families and friends. It includes case studies and diaries of people in recovery, tools for removing barriers to care, and information about the treatments suitable for self-injury.

Kettewell, C. (1999) *Skin game.* St. Martin's Press, Griffin, NY.
A memoir of self-injury. The author, an acclaimed author and journalist, engaged in a pattern of self-injury for many years, starting in early adolescence.

Levenkron, S. (1999) *Cutting: understanding and overcoming self-mutilation.* Norton Books, New York, NY.
This book is suitable for a range of audiences, including people who engage in self-injury, families and friends, and health professionals who wish to better understand the behavior. It explains the psychological motivations for nonsuicidal self-injury, common risk factors, and benefits of treatment.

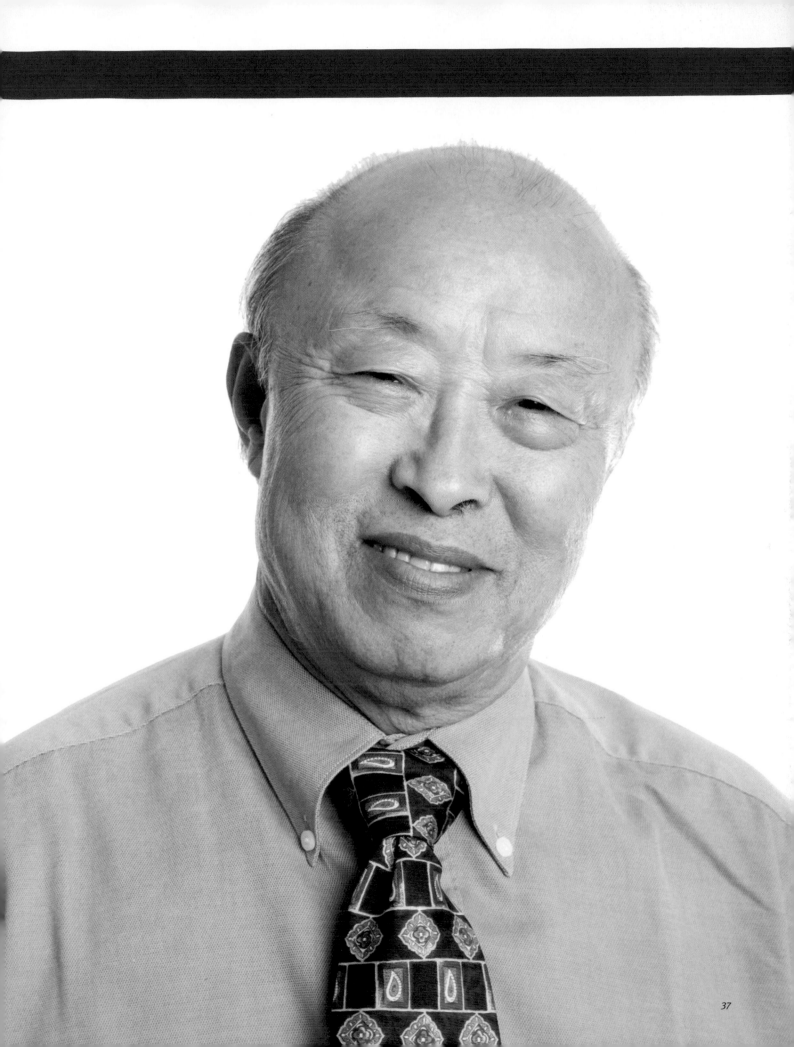

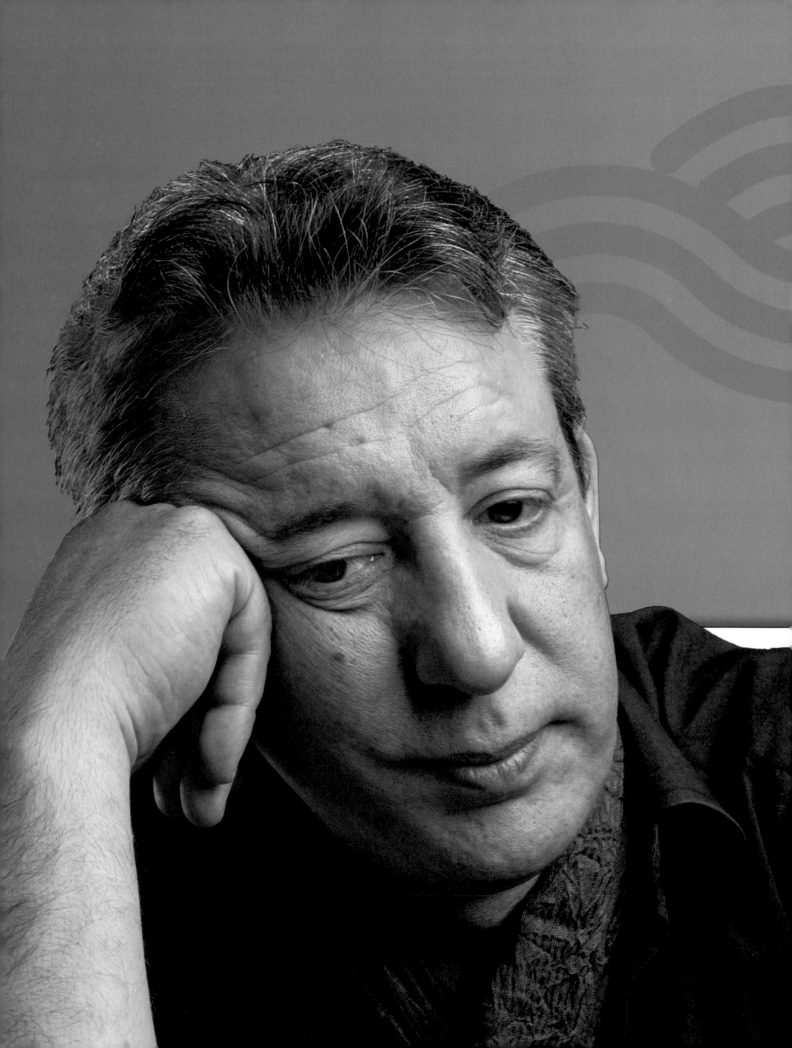

CHAPTER 4

Anxiety Disorders

What Is an Anxiety Disorder?

Everyone experiences anxiety at some time—anxiety can be quite useful in helping a person to avoid dangerous situations and motivate the solving of everyday problems. Anxiety can vary in severity from mild uneasiness to a terrifying panic attack. Anxiety also can vary in how long it lasts, from a few minutes to many years. An anxiety disorder differs from normal anxiety in the following ways:

- It is more intense.

- It is long lasting.

- It interferes with the person's work, activities, or relationships.

Approximately 19 percent of U.S. adults have an anxiety disorder[1] in a given year. Anxiety disorders tend to begin in childhood, adolescence, or early adulthood. The median age of onset is 11 years,[2] which means half the people have their first episode by this age. Anxiety disorders often occur with mood disorders and substance use disorder. Anxiety disorders are more common in females than in males.

Anxiety can show in a variety of ways: physical, psychological, and behavioral. General symptoms of anxiety can be found in anxiety disorders.

Symptoms of Anxiety[21]

PHYSICAL

>> **Cardiovascular:** pounding heart, chest pain, rapid heartbeat, flushing

>> **Respiratory:** hyperventilation, shortness of breath

>> **Neurological:** dizziness, headache, sweating, tingling, numbness

>> **Gastrointestinal:** choking, dry mouth, stomach pains, nausea, vomiting, diarrhea

>> **Musculoskeletal:** muscle aches and pains (especially neck, shoulders, and back), restlessness, tremors and shaking, inability to relax.

PSYCHOLOGICAL

Unrealistic and/or excessive fear and worry (about past and future events), mind racing or going blank, decreased concentration and memory, indecisiveness, irritability, impatience, anger, confusion, restlessness or feeling "on edge" or nervous, tiredness, sleep disturbance, vivid dreams.

BEHAVIORAL

Avoidance of situations, obsessive or compulsive behavior, distress in social situations, phobic behavior.

Types of Anxiety Disorders

There are many different types of anxiety disorders.[21] The main ones are phobic disorders, post-traumatic stress disorder, generalized anxiety disorder, panic disorder, and obsessive–compulsive disorder. The table below shows how common each of these is:

Percentage of American Adults with Anxiety Disorders in Any One Year [1,2,57]		
TYPE OF MENTAL DISORDER	**ADULTS**	**MEDIAN AGE OF ONSET**
Specific Phobia	9.1%	7 years
Social Phobia	7.1%	13 years
Post-Traumatic Stress Disorder	3.6%	23 years
Generalized Anxiety Disorder	2.7%	31 years
Panic Disorder	2.7%	24 years
Obsessive–Compulsive Disorder	1.2%	19 years
Agoraphobia (without panic)	0.9%	20 years
Any Anxiety Disorder	19.1%	11 years

Generalized Anxiety Disorder

The main symptoms of generalized anxiety disorder (GAD) are overwhelming, unfounded anxiety and worry (about things that may go wrong or one's inability to cope) accompanied by multiple physical and psychological symptoms of anxiety or tension occurring more days than not for at least 6 months. People with generalized anxiety disorder worry excessively about money, health, family, and work, even when there are no signs of trouble. The anxiety appears difficult to control. Other characteristics include an intolerance of uncertainty, belief that worry is a helpful way to deal with problems, and poor problem-solving skills. GAD can make it difficult for people to concentrate at school or work, function at home, and generally get on with their lives.

Panic Disorder

It is important to distinguish between a panic attack and a panic disorder. A panic attack is a sudden onset of intense apprehension, fear, or terror. These attacks begin suddenly and develop rapidly. This intense fear is inappropriate for the circumstances in which it is occurring. Other symptoms, many of which can appear similar to those of a heart attack, can include racing heart, sweating, shortness of breath, chest pain, dizziness, feeling detached from oneself, and fears of losing control. Once a person has had one of these attacks, they often fear another attack and may avoid places where attacks have occurred. The person may avoid exercise or other activities that may produce physical sensations similar to those of a panic attack.

Having a panic attack does not necessarily mean that a person will develop panic disorder. A person with a panic disorder experiences recurring panic attacks and, for at least 1 month, is persistently worried about possible future panic attacks and possible consequences of panic attacks, such as losing control or having a heart attack. Some people may develop panic disorder after only a few panic attacks, while others may experience many panic attacks without developing a panic disorder. Some people with panic disorder go on to develop agoraphobia, where they avoid places in fear of having a panic attack.

Phobic Disorders

A person with a phobic disorder avoids or restricts activities because of persistent and excessive fear. They may have an unreasonably strong fear of specific places, events, or objects and often avoid these completely.

>> **Agoraphobia** involves avoidance of situations where the person fears having a panic attack. The focus of his/her anxiety is that it will be difficult or embarrassing to get away from the place if a panic attack occurs or that there will be no one

present who can help. This leads to avoiding certain situations out of fear. Some may avoid only a few situations or places, such as crowds, shopping malls or other enclosed spaces, or driving. Others may avoid leaving home altogether.

>> **Social phobia** is the fear of any situation where public scrutiny may occur, usually with the fear of behaving in a way that is embarrassing or humiliating. Social phobia often develops in shy children as they move into adolescence. Commonly feared situations include speaking or eating in public, dating, and social events.

>> **Specific phobias** are phobias of specific objects or situations. The most common are spiders, bugs, mice, snakes, and heights. Other feared objects or situations include an animal, blood, injections, storms, driving, flying, or enclosed places. Because they involve specific situations or objects, these phobias are usually less disabling than agoraphobia and social phobia.

Acute Stress Disorder and Post-traumatic Stress Disorder

Acute stress disorder and post-traumatic stress disorder occur after a distressing or catastrophic event. Common examples include involvement in war, accidents (such as traffic or physical accidents), assault (including physical or sexual assault, mugging or robbery, or family violence), or witnessing a significant event. Mass traumatic events include terrorist attacks, mass shootings, and severe weather events (such as hurricane, tsunami, or forest fire).

In acute stress disorder, the person gets over the event within a month, whereas in post-traumatic stress disorder, the distress lasts longer. Some who experience acute stress disorder go on to develop post-traumatic stress disorder. A person is more likely to develop post-traumatic stress if the response to an event involves intense fear, helplessness, or horror.

A major symptom is reexperiencing the trauma. This can include recurrent dreams, flashbacks, intrusive memories, or unrest in situations that bring back memories of the original trauma.

There is also avoidance behavior, such as persistent avoidance of stimuli associated with the event, as well as emotional numbing, which may continue for months or years, and reduced interest in others and the outside world. Persistent symptoms of increased arousal also can occur, such as constant watchfulness, irritability, jumpiness, being easily startled, outbursts of rage, or insomnia.

For information on how to help someone who has experienced a traumatic event, see *First Aid for Adults Affected by Traumatic Events* and *First Aid for Children Affected by Traumatic Events*.

Obsessive–Compulsive Disorder

Obsessive–compulsive disorder is the least common anxiety disorder but can be very disabling. Obsessive thoughts and compulsive behaviors accompany feelings of anxiety. Obsessive thoughts are recurrent impulses and images that are experienced as intrusive, unwanted, and inappropriate and cause marked anxiety. Obsessive thoughts and impulses include fear of contamination, the need for symmetry and exactness, safety issues, sexual impulses, aggressive impulses, and religious preoccupation.

Compulsive behaviors are repetitive behaviors or mental acts that the person feels driven to perform to reduce anxiety. Common compulsions include washing, checking, repeating, ordering, counting, hoarding, or touching things over and over.

Mixed Anxiety, Depression, and Substance Abuse

Many people have anxiety problems that do not fit neatly into a particular type of disorder. It is common for people to have some features of several anxiety disorders. A person who experiences a high level of anxiety over a long period will often develop depression, so many have a mixture of anxiety and depression.

Substance abuse frequently occurs with anxiety disorders as a form of self-medication. Alcohol and other drug abuse can also lead to increased anxiety.

What Causes Anxiety Disorders?

Anxiety is mostly caused by perceived threats in the environment, but some people are more likely than others to react with anxiety when threatened. Those most at risk[58]

- Have a more sensitive emotional nature and tend to see the world as threatening

- Have a history of anxiety in childhood or adolescence, including marked shyness

- Are female

- Abuse alcohol

- Have had a traumatic experience.

Some family factors that increase risk are

- Difficult childhood (for example, experiencing physical, emotional, or sexual abuse, neglect, or overstrictness)

- Family background that involves poverty or lack of job skills

- Family history of anxiety disorders

- Parental alcohol problems

- Separation and divorce.

Anxiety symptoms also can result from

- Some medical conditions, including endocrine conditions such as hyperthyroidism, cardiac conditions such as arrhythmias, respiratory conditions such as chronic obstructive pulmonary disease and metabolic conditions such as vitamin B12 deficiency[21]

- Side effects of certain prescription drugs

- Intoxication with alcohol, amphetamines, caffeine, marijuana, cocaine, hallucinogens, and inhalants

- Withdrawal from alcohol, cocaine, sedatives, and antianxiety medications

Some develop ways of reducing anxiety that actually cause further problems. For example, people with phobias avoid anxiety-provoking situations. This avoidance reduces their anxiety in the short term, but can limit their lives in significant ways. Similarly, people with compulsions reduce their anxiety by repetitive acts such as frequent hand washing. These compulsions become problems in themselves. Some people will use drugs or alcohol to cope, which can increase anxiety in the long term.

Importance of Early Intervention for Anxiety Disorders

It is important that anxiety disorders are recognized and treated early. Anxiety disorders often develop in childhood and adolescence, and if not treated, the person is more likely to have a range of adverse outcomes later in life, such as depression, alcohol dependence, illicit drug dependence, suicide attempts, lowered educational achievement, and early parenthood.[58] Because of these long-term consequences, it is important that anxiety disorders are recognized early and people get appropriate professional help.

The Mental Health First Aid Action Plan for Anxiety Disorders

MENTAL HEALTH FIRST AID ACTION PLAN	
ACTION A	Assess for risk of suicide or harm
ACTION L	Listen nonjudgmentally
ACTION G	Give reassurance and information
ACTION E	Encourage appropriate professional help
ACTION E®	Encourage self-help and other support strategies

FACTS ON TRAUMATIC EVENTS[59]

A *traumatic event* is any incident perceived to be traumatic. Common examples include accidents (such as traffic or physical accidents), assault (including physical or sexual assault, mugging or robbery, or family violence), or witnessing something terrible. Mass traumatic events include terrorist attacks, mass shootings, and severe weather events (such as hurricane, tsunami, forest fire).

Trauma isn't always a single event; it can occur over time. Common examples of recurring trauma include sexual, physical, or emotional abuse; torture; and bullying in the schoolyard or workplace. Sometimes the memories of a traumatic event suddenly or unexpectedly return weeks, months, or even years afterwards. In either case, Mental Health First Aid guidelines can be used when the first aider becomes aware of an emerging issue.

It is important to know that people differ in how they react to traumatic events:

- One person may perceive an event as deeply traumatic, while another may not.

- Particular types of trauma affect some individuals more than others.

- A history of trauma may make some people more susceptible to later traumatic events, while others become more resilient.

ACTION A: Assess for risk of suicide or harm

The technique that is helpful for assessing risk in someone with anxiety is similar to that used with someone experiencing depression; see Chapter 3. The key points are as follows:

- Approach the person about the concerns regarding their anxiety.

- Find a suitable time and space where you both feel comfortable.

- If the person does not initiate a conversation with you about how they are feeling, you can begin a dialogue.

- Respect the person's privacy and confidentiality.

Crises that may be associated with anxiety include

- *An extreme level of anxiety* (this may be a *panic attack* or a *reaction to a recent traumatic event* in a person's life)

- *Suicidal thoughts and behaviors*

- Engaging in *nonsuicidal self-injury*

*If you determine the person is **not in crisis**, you can ask how they are feeling, how long they have been feeling that way, and move on to Action L.*

Symptoms of a Panic Attack[21]

A panic attack is a distinct episode of high anxiety with fear or discomfort. It develops abruptly and has its peak within 10 minutes. During the attack, several of the following symptoms are present:

- Palpitations, pounding heart, rapid heart rate

- Sweating

- Trembling and shaking

- Shortness of breath, sensations of choking or smothering

- Chest pain or discomfort

- Abdominal distress or nausea

- Dizziness, light-headedness, feeling faint or unsteady

- Feelings of unreality or being detached from oneself

- Fear of losing control or "going crazy"

- Fear of dying

- Numbness or tingling

- Chills or hot flashes.

Suicidal thoughts may not be as evident as extreme anxiety, but there is a risk of suicide in anxiety disorders. Therefore, in any interaction with a person, be alert to any warning signs of suicide. For advice on what to look for and how to ask the person about suicidal feelings, refer to Chapter 3.

The risk of suicide in people with anxiety disorders is not as high as for some other mental disorders.[44] However, the risk increases if the person has a concurrent mood or substance use disorder.

Let the person know that you are concerned and are willing to help.

>> If it appears the person is having a *panic attack*, see *First Aid for Panic Attacks*.

>> If the person is *distressed after experiencing a traumatic event*, see *First Aid for Traumatic Events*.

>> If there is concern about *suicidal thoughts*, see *First Aid for Suicidal Thoughts and Behaviors*.

If you have serious concerns, call 911 or the National Suicide Prevention Lifeline at 1-800-273-TALK (8255).

>> If the person is engaging in *nonsuicidal self-injury*, see *First Aid for Nonsuicidal Self-Injury*.

ACTION L: Listen nonjudgmentally

- Engage the person in discussing their feelings.

- Listen to the person without judging.

- Pay close attention to what the person says.

- Reflect or restate what the person has said.

- Ask clarifying questions to show that you want to understand.

- Maintain comfortable eye contact.

- Use minimal prompts, such as "I see" and "ah."

- Be patient and do not interrupt.

- Allow silences.

- Maintain an open body position.

- Do not be critical of the person.

- Do not express frustration at the person for having such symptoms.

- Do not give flippant or unhelpful advice such as "pull yourself together."

- Avoid confrontation unless necessary to prevent harmful acts.

See Action L in Chapter 3 for more tips on nonjudgmental listening.

ACTION G: Give reassurance and information

The assurance and information helpful to someone with troublesome anxiety is similar to that given to someone with depression. You can support the person in the following ways:

- Treat the person with respect and dignity.

- Do not blame the person for the illness.

- Have realistic expectations for the person.

- Offer consistent emotional support and understanding.

- Give the person hope for recovery.

- Provide practical help.

- Offer information.

See Action G in Chapter 3 for more advice about giving reassurance and information.

WHAT ISN'T SUPPORTIVE?

It is important to know that recovery from anxiety disorders requires facing situations that can provoke anxiety. Avoiding such situations can slow recovery and make anxiety worse. Sometimes, family and friends think they are being supportive by facilitating the person's avoidance of anxiety-provoking situations, but this can inadvertently slow recovery.

Other actions that are not supportive include dismissing fears as trivial, for example, by saying, *That is nothing to be afraid of*, telling them to *toughen up* or *don't be so weak*, or using a patronizing tone of voice.

ACTION E: Encourage appropriate professional help

Many people with anxiety disorders do not realize there are treatments that can help. In the United States, only 42 percent of the people who had an anxiety disorder in the past year received treatment for their problem.[30] Even when people finally seek help, a delay of 10 years or more is not unusual.[31] These delays can cause serious consequences in the person's life, limiting social and occupational opportunities and increasing the risk for depression and drug and alcohol problems.

DISCUSS OPTIONS FOR SEEKING PROFESSIONAL HELP

Offer the person help to manage their feelings. If help is needed, then respond as follows:

- Discuss appropriate professional help and effective treatment options.

- Encourage the person to use these options.

- Offer to help them seek out these options.

- Encourage the person not to give up seeking appropriate professional help.

PROFESSIONALS WHO CAN HELP

A variety of health professionals can provide help to a person with anxiety disorders:

- Primary care physicians

- Mental health professionals

- Certified peer specialists

- Psychiatrists.

More information about how these professionals can help is available in Chapter 1.

If the person is uncertain about what to do, encourage consultation with a primary care physician first, as the physician can check for an underlying physical health cause for this anxiety and refer the person to the appropriate specialized help.

Treatments Available for Anxiety Disorders

Research shows that both medication and cognitive behavioral therapy (CBT) are effective treatments.[60]

MEDICATION

Different types of antidepressants have been found to be effective in treating specific anxiety disorders. Antianxiety medications (benzodiazepines) also are effective but should be restricted to short-term use because of concerns about possible side effects of dependency, sedation, rebound anxiety, and memory impairment.

COGNITIVE BEHAVIORAL THERAPY

Various psychological therapies are used for anxiety disorders, but CBT has, by far, the strongest evidence for effectiveness. CBT may include

- Education about self-managing the anxiety

- Problem solving where the person and clinician work together to identify problems and generate and implement solutions

- Exposure–response therapy to feared situations or symptoms aiming to overcome the avoidance behavior

- Cognitive restructuring focusing on identifying automatic negative thoughts and considering alternative ways of thinking

- Emotion regulation through relaxation and learning detachment from strong anxiety

- Social skills strategies to use in anxiety-provoking situations

- Relapse prevention plan for coping with anxiety if it returns.

A person can undertake a program of CBT in a number of different ways. CBT can be delivered by a therapist working one to one or in a group of people with similar problems or through systematically working through a self-help book or a self-help website. Useful self-help books and websites are listed at the end of this chapter.

WHAT IF THE PERSON DOESN'T WANT HELP?

The person may not want to seek professional help, so you might probe to discover the reason. For example, the person might be concerned about finances or about not having a doctor they like. You may be able to help the person overcome the worry about seeking help. If the person still doesn't want help after you have explored the reasons, let them know that if they change their mind about seeking help, they can contact you. Respect the person's right not to seek help unless you believe they are at risk of harming self or others.

ACTION E: Encourage self-help and other support strategies

OTHER PEOPLE WHO CAN HELP

Encourage the person to consider other available support, such as family, friends, faith communities, or people who have also experienced troublesome anxiety (peer supporters). There is also evidence that mutual support groups may be helpful for people with depression and anxiety problems.[14]

SELF-HELP STRATEGIES

People who are troubled with anxiety frequently use self-help strategies. The person's ability and desire to use self-help will depend on their interests and the severity of their symptoms. Therefore, do not be overly forceful when trying to encourage the person to use self-help strategies.

Therapies with scientific evidence for effectiveness with anxiety disorders include [61, 62]

- Relaxation training

- Exercise

- Self-help books based on CBT

- Meditation.

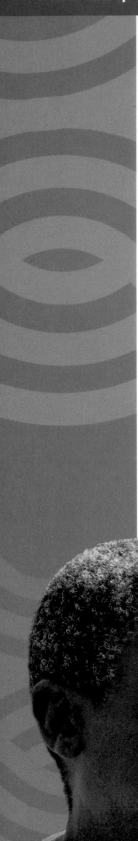

Helpful Resources

WEBSITES

Anxiety Disorders Association of America

www.adaa.org

ADAA promotes the early diagnosis, treatment, and cure of anxiety disorders.

Anxiety Panic Attack Resource Site

www.anxietypanic.com

This site provides information pertaining to a variety of treatments and resources on anxiety. The site also provides questionnaires, links to treatment resources, a message board, and lists helpful publications.

Benson-Henry Institute for Mind Body Medicine

www.massgeneral.org/bhi/store/

The Benson-Henry Institute for Mind Body Medicine at Massachusetts General Hospital has an online store providing CDs, DVDs, and books on relaxation techniques.

E-couch

ecouch.anu.edu.au

The E-couch website provides information about emotional problems (including depression and anxiety disorders)—what causes them, how to prevent them, and how to treat them. It also provides a set of evidence-based online interventions designed to equip the user with strategies to improve mood and emotional state, along with a workbook to track progress and record experiences.

Freedom From Fear

www.freedomfromfear.org

The Freedom From Fear website provides information, screening tools, and other resources on many types of anxiety disorders.

Mental Health America

www.mentalhealthamerica.net

Visit Mental Health America's site for information on mental health, getting help, and taking action.

National Council for Behavioral Health

www.TheNationalCouncil.org

To locate mental health and addictions treatment facilities in your community, use the Find a Provider feature on the National Council's website.

National Institute of Mental Health

www.nimh.nih.gov

The website for the National Institute of Mental Health has a wealth of information on anxiety disorders.

Obsessive–Compulsive Foundation

www.ocfoundation.org

The Obsessive-Compulsive Foundation website includes information about obsessive–compulsive disorder, including information about effective treatments, how to find a health professional who has experience treating the disorder, and links to other websites.

BOOKS

GENERAL BOOKS

Bourne, E. J. (2010) *The anxiety and phobia workbook.* (5th ed.). Oakland, CA: New Harbinger Publications, Inc.
This is a self-help book based on cognitive behavioral therapy (CBT).

Marks, I. (2001) *Living with fear.* McGraw-Hill Education, Berkshire, England.
This book is based on CBT. It includes a very useful chapter on self-help for fears and anxiety. Research has shown that people with phobias who follow the instructions in this chapter improve as much as people treated by a professional.

PANIC BOOKS

Antony, M. M., and McCabe, R. (2004) *10 simple solutions to panic: how to overcome panic attacks, calm physical symptoms, and reclaim your life.* New Harbinger Publications, Oakland, CA.
This small-format self-help book is based on CBT principles and may help people who experience panic attacks. The focus is on thinking realistically about future attacks rather than worrying about them.

Zuercher-White, E. (1998) *An end to panic: breakthrough techniques for overcoming panic disorder.* New Harbinger Publications, Oakland, CA.
This self-help workbook is based on CBT principles and may help people who experience panic attacks, panic disorder, and agoraphobia.

PHOBIA BOOKS

Antony, M. M. and McCabe, R. (2005) *Overcoming animal & insect phobias: how to conquer fear of dogs, snakes, rodents, bees, spiders & more.* New Harbinger Publications, Oakland, CA.
This book is part of the "I Can Do It" Series. It uses a self-help approach to graded exposure, a form of CBT, for overcoming animal and insect phobias.

Antony, M. M. and Watling, M. (2006) *Overcoming medical phobias: how to conquer fear of blood, needles, doctors, and dentists.* New Harbinger Publications, Oakland, CA.
Medical phobias can lead to significant medical problems, as individuals may resist seeking medical help for emerging problems and emergencies. This book is part of the "I Can Do It" Series. It uses a self-help approach to graded exposure, a form of CBT, for overcoming medical phobias.

SOCIAL ANXIETY BOOKS

Antony, M. M. (2004) *10 simple solutions to shyness: how to overcome shyness, social anxiety, & fear of public speaking.* New Harbinger Publications, Oakland, CA.
This small-format book is an excellent accompaniment to the book listed below. Based on the principles of CBT, it may be useful not only to individuals with a clinical disorder but also to those who are nervous in social situations or speaking in public.

Antony, M. M., & Swinson, P. R. (2008)
The shyness and social anxiety workbook: proven step-by-step techniques for overcoming your fears. (2nd ed.). Oakland, CA: New Harbinger Publications, Inc.
This large-format self-help workbook uses the principles of CBT to help people overcome shyness and social phobia.

Stein, M. B., & Walker, J. R. (2002) *Triumph over shyness: conquering shyness & social anxiety*. New York, NY: McGraw-Hill.
This self-help book is copublished and endorsed by the Anxiety Disorders Association of America. It may be useful for people with social phobia but also those who struggle with nonclinical shyness. A range of approaches is used.

OBSESSIVE–COMPULSIVE DISORDER BOOKS

Foa, E. B. and Wilson, R. (2001) *Stop obsessing: how to overcome your obsessions and compulsions*. Revised edition. Bantam Books, New York, NY.
A CBT-based self-help manual for overcoming OCD. Readers are encouraged to tailor a CBT program to target specific obsessions and compulsions. It also includes self-tests and case studies from the authors' significant clinical backgrounds.

The following four books are a suite of self-help workbooks that focus on practical strategies for overcoming specific types of OCD. By selecting the workbook that focuses on the main compulsive symptom (checking, washing, or hoarding) and then adding the workbook on obsessions, an individual can create his own CBT program for overcoming OCD.

Munford, P. (2004) *Overcoming compulsive checking: free your mind from OCD*. New Harbinger Publications, Oakland, CA.

Munford, P. (2004) *Overcoming compulsive washing: free your mind from OCD*. New Harbinger Publications, Oakland, CA.

Neviroglu, F. and Bubrick, J. (2004) *Overcoming compulsive hoarding: why you save and how you can stop*. New Harbinger Publications, Oakland, CA.

Purdon, C. and Clark, D. A. (2005) *Overcoming obsessive thoughts: how to gain control of your OCD*. New Harbinger Publications, Oakland, CA.

HELP LINES

American Psychiatric Association Answer Center
1-888-35-PSYCH (1-888-357-7924)
Live operators, available from 8:30 a.m. to 6 p.m., Eastern time, refer you to local board-certified psychiatrists.

American Psychological Association Public Education Line
1-800-964-2000
Follow the automated instructions and press the number 1. Then an operator refers you to local board-certified psychologists.

SUPPORT GROUPS

American Self-Help Group Clearinghouse

www.mentalhelp.net/selfhelp/

This searchable database contains more than 1,100 self-help and caregiver support groups, including many for anxiety disorders. Also listed are local self-help clearinghouses worldwide, research studies, information on starting face-to-face and online groups, and a registry for persons interested in starting national or international self-help groups.

National Alliance on Mental Illness

www.nami.org

On the home page, click on "Find Support."

Recovery International

www.recovery-inc.com

On the home page, click on "Find A Meeting" to find the next Recovery International meeting in your area.

Recovery International, a Chicago-based self-help mental health organization, sponsors weekly group peer-led meetings across the United States, as well as telephone and Internet-based meetings.

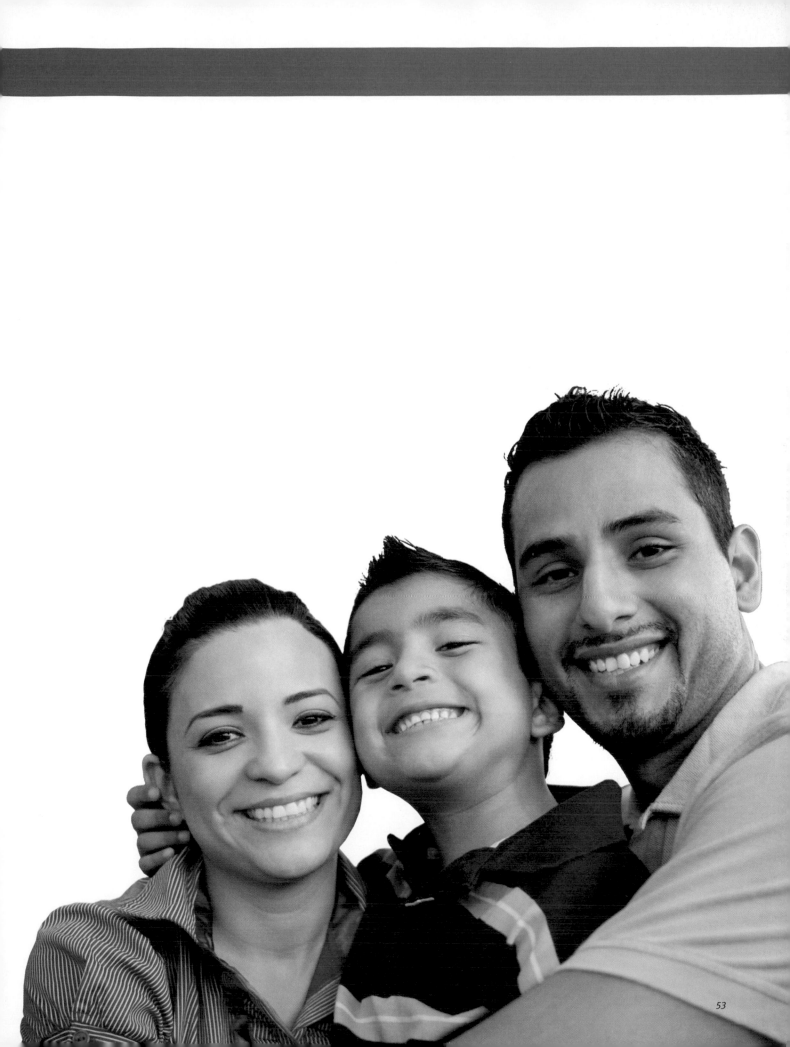

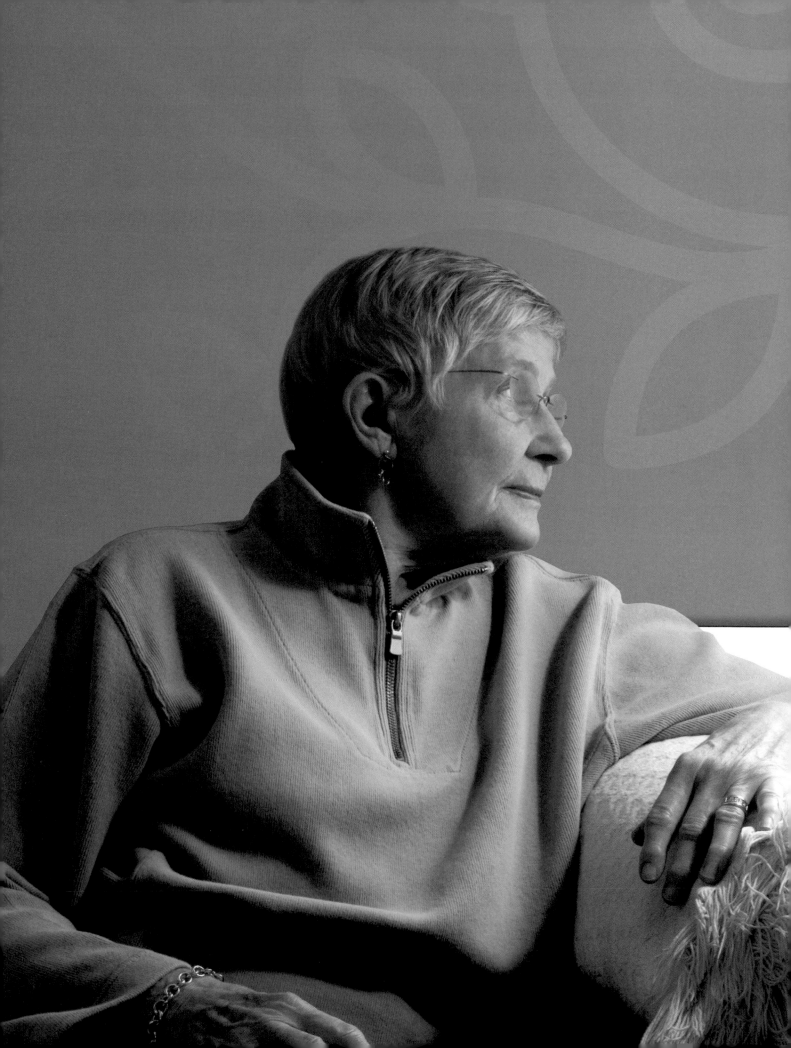

CHAPTER 5

Psychosis

What Is Psychosis?

Psychosis is a general term used to describe a mental health problem in which a person has lost some contact with reality, resulting in severe disturbances in thinking, emotion, and behavior. Psychosis can severely disrupt a person's relationships, work, and usual activities. Self-care can be difficult to initiate or maintain.

Disorders in which psychosis may occur are less common than other mental disorders. There are numerous disorders in which a person can experience psychosis, including schizophrenia, bipolar disorder, psychotic depression, schizoaffective disorder, drug-induced psychosis, and delirium.

People usually experience psychosis in episodes. An episode can involve the following phases, which can vary in length:

>> **Premorbid** (at-risk phase)—the person does not experience symptoms but has risk factors for developing psychosis

>> **Prodromal** (becoming unwell phase)—the person has some changes in emotions, motivation, thinking, and perception or behavior, as described below

>> **Acute** (psychotic phase)—the person is unwell with psychotic symptoms such as delusions, hallucinations, disorganized thinking, and reduction in ability to maintain social relationships, work, or study

>> **Recovery**—an individual journey to attain a level of well-being

>> **Relapse**—the person may have only one episode or may have additional episodes.

Common Symptoms When Psychosis Is Developing[63]

CHANGES IN EMOTION AND MOTIVATION
Depression; anxiety; irritability; suspiciousness; blunted, flat, or inappropriate emotion; change in appetite; reduced energy and motivation.

CHANGES IN THINKING AND PERCEPTION
Difficulties with concentration or attention; a sense of alteration, such as the feeling that they or others have changed or are acting differently in some way; odd ideas; an unusual perceptual experience, such as reduction or greater intensity of smell, sound, or color.

CHANGES IN BEHAVIOR
Sleep disturbances, social isolation or withdrawal, reduced ability to carry out work or social roles.

Although these signs and symptoms may not be very dramatic on their own, when they are considered together, they may suggest that something is not quite right. It is important not to ignore or dismiss such warning signs, even if they appear gradually or are unclear. Do not assume the person is going through a phase or misusing alcohol or other drugs or that symptoms will go away on their own.

Signs and symptoms of psychosis may vary from person to person and can change over time. It is also important to consider the spiritual and cultural context of the person's behaviors, as what is interpreted as a symptom of psychosis in one culture may be considered normal in another.

People experiencing early stages of psychosis often go undiagnosed for a year or more before receiving treatment. A major reason for this is that psychosis often begins in late adolescence or early adulthood and the early signs and symptoms involve behaviors and emotions that are common in this age group.

Many young people will have experienced some of these symptoms without developing a psychosis. Others showing these symptoms will eventually be diagnosed as having a psychotic disorder.

Types of Disorders in which Psychosis Can Occur

Schizophrenia

The most common disorder in which psychosis is a feature is schizophrenia. Contrary to common belief, schizophrenia does not mean "split personality." The term "schizophrenia" comes from the Greek word for "fractured mind" and refers to changes in mental function where thoughts and perceptions become disordered.

The major symptoms of schizophrenia include the following:

>> **Delusions:** False beliefs of persecution, guilt, having a special mission, or being under outside control. Although the delusions may seem bizarre to others, they are very real to the person experiencing them.

>> **Hallucinations:** Most commonly involve hearing voices, but can also involve seeing, feeling, tasting, or smelling things. These are perceived as very real by the person but are not actually there. Hallucinations can be frightening, especially voices saying negative comments. The person may hear more than one voice or additionally experience many different types of hallucinations. Because delusions and hallucinations seem so real, it is common for people with schizophrenia to be unaware they are ill.

>> **Thinking difficulties:** Difficulties in concentration, memory, and ability to plan, making it difficult for the person to reason, communicate, and complete daily tasks.

>> **Loss of drive:** Lack of motivation even for self-care. It is not laziness.

>> **Blunted emotions:** The person seems oblivious to the things around them and often reacts inappropriately. Examples include speaking in a monotone, lack of facial expressions or gestures, and lack of eye contact.

>> **Social withdrawal:** The person may withdraw from contact with others, even family and close friends. There may be a number of factors that lead to this withdrawal, such as loss of drive, delusions that cause fear of interacting, difficulty concentrating on conversations, and loss of social skills.

Schizophrenia affects approximately 1.4 million Americans each year (0.45%).[23] Most experience their first episode of schizophrenia between ages 15 and 25.[64] Schizophrenia knows no racial, cultural, or economic boundaries. It affects males more than females, and males tend to develop it earlier.[65] The onset of illness may be rapid, with symptoms developing over several weeks, or it may be slow, developing over months or years. Approximately one third of people who develop schizophrenia have only one episode and fully recover, another third have multiple episodes but feel well in between episodes, and a third have a lifelong illness.[66]

Bipolar Disorder[67]

People with bipolar disorder have extreme mood swings. They can experience periods of depression, periods of mania, and long periods of normal mood in between. The time between these different episodes can vary greatly from person to person. It is not unusual for people with this disorder to become psychotic during depressive or manic episodes.[33, 34]

The *depression* experienced by a person with bipolar disorder has some or all of the symptoms of depression listed in Chapter 3.

A person experiencing *mania* will have some of the following symptoms:

>> **Increased energy and overactivity**

>> **Elevated mood:** The person will feel high, happy, full of energy, on the top of the world, and invincible.

>> **Need less sleep than usual:** The person can go for days with very little sleep.

>> **Irritability:** This may occur if others disagree with unrealistic plans or ideas.

>> **Rapid thinking and speech:** The person may talk too much and too fast and keep changing topics.

>> **Lack of inhibitions:** The person may disregard risk, spend money extravagantly, or be very sexually active.

>> **Grandiose delusions:** These involve very inflated self-esteem, such as a belief that the person is superhuman, especially talented, or an important religious figure.

>> **Lack of insight:** The person is so convinced that their manic delusions are real that they do not realize they are ill.

It can take people with bipolar disorder a long time to be diagnosed correctly because the person must have had episodes of both depression and mania. It affects 2.6 percent of adults in any one year.[1] Fifty percent of people have their first episode by age 25[2], and males and females are equally affected. See Chapter 3 for other information about bipolar disorder.

Psychotic Depression

Sometimes depression can be so intense it causes psychotic symptoms. For example, the person may experience delusions involving guilt, severe physical illness, or hopelessness.

Schizoaffective Disorder

Schizoaffective disorder describes a condition where symptoms of a mood disorder and symptoms of schizophrenia are both present. Sometimes it is difficult to tell the difference between schizophrenia and bipolar disorder, as the person has symptoms of both illnesses.

Drug-Induced Psychosis

Psychosis can be brought on by intoxication or withdrawal from drugs. The symptoms usually appear quickly and last a short time (from a few hours to a few days) until the effects of the drugs wear off. The most common symptoms are visual hallucinations, disorientation, and memory problems. Both legal and illegal drugs can contribute to a psychotic episode, including marijuana (cannabis), alcohol, cocaine, amphetamine (speed), hallucinogens, inhalants, opioids, sedatives, hypnotics, and anxiolytics.[21]

What Causes Psychosis?

It is believed psychosis is caused by a combination of factors, including genetics, biochemistry, and stress. Biological factors could be genetic vulnerability, changes in the brain, or a dysfunction in the neurotransmitters in the brain. Stress or drug abuse may trigger psychotic symptoms in vulnerable people.

Risk Factors for Schizophrenia[68]

>> **Having a close relative with schizophrenia.** For someone with a parent or sibling with schizophrenia, the risk is around 10% to 15%. Although the risk is higher, it is important to note that 85% to 90% will not develop schizophrenia.

>> **Male gender.** Males are more likely to develop schizophrenia and tend to have an earlier age of onset.

>> **Urban living.** People who are born and grow up in urban areas are at higher risk than those from rural areas. The reason is unknown but could be related to differences in the health of mothers during pregnancy, marijuana use, or social stressors.

>> **Migration.** Immigrants and children of immigrants have increased risk. The reason is unknown, but social stress from feeling like an outsider could be a factor.

>> **Social stress.** Social stressors can trigger the onset of schizophrenia.

>> **Marijuana use.** Marijuana use during adolescence increases risk, particularly in people who have other risk factors.[69]

>> **Events during pregnancy.** Infections in the mother in the first and second trimesters of pregnancy have been linked with higher incidence. A possible explanation is that the mother's immune response interferes with the brain development of the fetus.

Severe nutritional deficiency and very stressful life events during pregnancy might also increase risk.

>> **Birth complications.** A range of complications is associated with double the risk, perhaps because of lack of oxygen (hypoxia) to the infant's brain.

>> **Birth in winter or spring.** Birth during the late winter or early spring is associated with 5 percent to 10 percent greater risk. The explanation is not known but may be related to infection, malnutrition, or risk of genetic mutation.

>> **Older age of father.** Older age at the time of conception roughly doubles the risk. The explanation is not known but may be related to impaired sperm and genetic mutation.

In persons with schizophrenia, the brain undergoes biochemical changes. One of the major known changes is to the neurotransmitter dopamine.[70] Antipsychotic medications used for schizophrenia work by altering dopamine levels in the brain.

Risk Factors for Bipolar Disorder[71]

The causes of bipolar disorder are not fully understood. However, the following factors are believed to be involved:

>> **Having a close relative with bipolar disorder.** This is the most important risk factor known. Someone with a parent or sibling affected has around a 9 percent risk.[72] While this is an increased risk, it means that more than 90 percent of people with an affected relative will not develop the disorder.

No other risk factors are firmly established. However, there is some research supporting the following:

>> **Pregnancy and obstetric complications.** These complications may affect the developing brain of the fetus or infant.

>> **Birth in winter or spring.** This may reflect risk to the fetus from infections or other events that vary by season.

>> **Social situation.** People who develop bipolar disorder are more likely to have lower income, be unemployed and single, and live in urban areas. However, these factors may be consequences of the early changes produced by bipolar disorder rather than causes.

>> **Recent stressful life events.** Stressful events are more common in the six months before onset of an episode of bipolar disorder than in people in general.

>> **Recent childbirth.** Women appear to be at increased risk in the months following childbirth.

>> **Brain injuries.** Brain injury before age 10 may increase risk.

>> **Multiple sclerosis.** People with multiple sclerosis may have increased risk.

Similar to schizophrenia, the risk factors for bipolar disorder can lead to biochemical changes in the brain, which produce mania and depression.

Importance of Early Intervention for Psychosis

Early intervention for people with psychosis is most important. Research has shown the longer the delay between the onset of psychosis and start of treatment, the less likely the person is to recover.[27] Other consequences of delayed treatment include[63]

- Poorer long-term functioning

- Increased risk of depression and suicide

- Slower psychological maturation and slower uptake of adult responsibilities

- Strain on relationships with friends and family and subsequent loss of social supports

- Disruption of study and employment

- Increased use of drugs and alcohol

- Loss of self-esteem and confidence

- Greater chance of problems with the law.

The Mental Health First Aid Action Plan for Psychosis

MENTAL HEALTH FIRST AID ACTION PLAN	
ACTION A	Assess for risk of suicide or harm
ACTION L	Listen nonjudgmentally
ACTION G	Give reassurance and information
ACTION E	Encourage appropriate professional help
ACTION E®	Encourage self-help and other support strategies

ACTION A: Assess for risk of suicide or harm[73]

People developing psychosis will often not reach out for help. Someone experiencing profound and frightening changes such as symptoms of psychosis will often try to keep it a secret. If you are concerned about someone, approach the person in a caring and nonjudgmental manner to discuss your concerns. Let the person know you are concerned and want to help. The person might not trust you or might be afraid of being perceived as "different" and therefore may not be open with you. If possible, approach the person privately about their experiences in a place that is free of distractions. Try to tailor your approach and interaction to the way the person is behaving. For example, if the person is suspicious and is avoiding eye contact, be sensitive to this and give him or her the space they need. Do not touch the person without permission. If they are unwilling, do not try to force them to talk about their experiences. Rather, let them know that you will be available if they would like to talk in the future. State the specific behaviors you are concerned about, and do not speculate about the person's diagnosis. It is important to allow the person to talk about his or her experiences and beliefs if he or she wants to. As far as possible, let the person set the pace and style of the interaction. Recognize the person might be frightened by his or her thoughts and feelings.

FACTS ON ACUTE PSYCHOSIS

A person who experiences psychosis has difficulty distinguishing what is real and what is not. Psychosis can occur as part of a number of mental disorders such as schizophrenia or bipolar disorder or when a person is intoxicated with a drug. In acute psychosis, the person will have severe symptoms such as delusions, hallucinations, very disorganized thinking, and odd behaviors. They may be unable to care for themselves appropriately. The person's behavior will be disruptive or disturbing to others, prompting them to seek assistance for the person's symptoms.[74]

FACTS ON THE RISK OF HARM AND PSYCHOSIS

Disorders in which psychosis can occur involve a high risk of suicide. Approximately 5 percent of people with schizophrenia complete suicide.[75] About 10 percent to 20 percent of individuals with bipolar disorder take their own life.

The main factors in assessing suicide risk in people experiencing symptoms of psychosis are[76, 77]

- Depression

- Suicidal thoughts, threats, or behavior

- Previous suicide attempt

- Poor adherence to treatment

- Fears of the impact of the illness on mental functioning

- Drug misuse.

A very small percentage of people experiencing psychosis may threaten violence.[78] People with mental disorders are often portrayed in the media as unpredictable, violent, or dangerous. However, the vast majority of people with mental disorders are not dangerous to others. Only a small proportion (up to 10 percent) of violence in society is due to mental illness.[79, 80] Depression and anxiety disorders have little or no association with violent behavior towards others. However, there is an increased risk of violence for people who experience substance use disorders, personality disorders, or psychosis.[81] The use of alcohol or other drugs has a stronger association with violence than do mental disorders. Many crimes are associated with people who have been using alcohol or other drugs.

There are two main crises associated with psychosis:

- The person is *at risk of harm to self or others* because they are acting upon delusions or hallucinations.

- The person has *suicidal thoughts and behaviors*.

Suicidal thoughts may not be as evident as aggression or risks of other harm and may require further interaction to assess risk. Further information on what to look for and how to ask the person if they are feeling suicidal can be found under Action A in Chapter 3.

If you have no concerns that the person is in crisis, you can ask him or her about how he or she is feeling and how long those feelings have lasted and move on to another Action.

Let the person know that you are concerned about them and are willing to help.

- If there is concern about *suicidal thoughts*, see *First Aid for Suicidal Thoughts and Behaviors*.

  If you have serious concerns, call 911 or the National Suicide Prevention Lifeline at 1-800-273-TALK (8255).

- If there is risk of *harm to self or others*, refer to *First Aid for Acute Psychosis* and also *First Aid for Aggressive Behavior*.

ACTION L: Listen nonjudgmentally

The person may be behaving and talking differently due to symptoms of psychosis. They may also find it difficult to tell what is real from what is not. Try to

- Understand the symptoms for what they are

- Empathize with how the person feels about his or her beliefs and experiences.

Try **not** to

- Confront the person

- Criticize or blame

- Take delusional comments personally

- Use sarcasm

- Use patronizing statements

- State any judgments about the content of those beliefs and experiences.

See Action L in Chapter 3 for more tips on nonjudgmental listening.

DEALING WITH DELUSIONS AND HALLUCINATIONS

It is important to recognize that delusions (false beliefs) and hallucinations (perceiving things that are not real) seem real to the person. Do not

- Dismiss, minimize, or argue with the person about their delusions or hallucinations

- Act alarmed, horrified, or embarrassed by the person's delusions or hallucinations

- Laugh at the person's symptoms of psychosis

- Encourage or inflame the person's paranoia, if the person exhibits paranoid behavior.

You can respond to the person's delusions without agreeing with them by saying something like, "That must be horrible for you" or "I can see that you are upset."

DEALING WITH COMMUNICATION DIFFICULTIES

People experiencing symptoms of psychosis are often unable to think or speak clearly. Ways to deal with communication difficulties include

- Responding to disorganized speech by communicating in an uncomplicated and clear manner

- Repeating things if necessary

- Being patient and allowing plenty of time for the person to process the information and respond to what you have said

- Being aware that it does not mean that the person is not feeling anything, even if the person is showing a limited range of feelings

- Not assuming the person cannot understand what you are saying, even if his or her response is limited.

ACTION G: Give reassurance and information

TREAT THE PERSON WITH RESPECT AND DIGNITY

Respect the person's autonomy while considering the extent to which he or she can make decisions for himself or herself. Respect the person's privacy and confidentiality unless you are concerned the person is at risk of harming himself or herself or others. Be honest when interacting with the person.

OFFER CONSISTENT EMOTIONAL SUPPORT AND UNDERSTANDING

Reassure them that you are there to help and support them and that you want to keep them safe.

GIVE THE PERSON HOPE FOR RECOVERY

Convey a message of hope by assuring them that help is available and things can get better.

PROVIDE PRACTICAL HELP

Try to find out what type of assistance they need by asking what will help them to feel safe and in control. If possible, offer the person choices of how you can help so that he or she is in control. Do not make promises you cannot keep. This can create an atmosphere of distrust and add to the person's distress.

OFFER INFORMATION

When a person is in a psychotic state, it is usually difficult and inappropriate to give information about psychosis. When the person is more lucid and in touch with reality, you could ask if he or she would like some information about psychosis. If they do want some information, it is important that you give them resources that are accurate and appropriate to their situation.

ACTION E: Encourage appropriate professional help

DISCUSS OPTIONS FOR SEEKING PROFESSIONAL HELP

Treatments and other supports available for psychosis are listed below. You could ask the person if they have felt this way before and, if so, what they have done in the past that has been helpful. If the person decides to seek professional help, make sure they are supported both emotionally and practically in accessing services. If the person does seek help, and either of you lack confidence in the medical advice received, seek a second opinion from another medical or mental health professional.

PROFESSIONALS WHO CAN HELP

A variety of health professionals can provide help to a person with psychosis. They are

- Primary care physicians

- Mental health professionals

- Certified peer specialists

- Psychiatrists.

More information about how these professionals can help is available in Chapter 1.

TREATMENTS AVAILABLE FOR PSYCHOSIS

The pattern of recovery from psychosis varies from person to person. Some people recover quickly with little intervention. Others may benefit from support over a longer period. Recovery from the first episode usually takes a number of months. If symptoms remain or return, the recovery process may be prolonged. Some people experience a difficult period lasting months or even years before effective management of further episodes of psychosis is achieved. Most people recover from psychosis and lead satisfying and productive lives. There is a range of treatments that have good evidence of effectively treating psychosis.

SCHIZOPHRENIA TREATMENTS[82]

In the past, people with schizophrenia were considered to have chronic illnesses with no hope of recovery. It is now known that people who get proper treatment can lead productive and fulfilling lives. In fact, research has demonstrated that recovery is possible with medication and psychosocial rehabilitation programs.

People with schizophrenia and other disorders in which psychosis can occur need to be regarded with optimism for a good outcome. They need to live in a stable and secure social environment. This includes a pleasant home environment, support from family and friends, an adequate income, and a meaningful role in society.[83] There is evidence that the following specific treatments help people with schizophrenia:

>> **Antipsychotic medications.** These are effective for psychotic symptoms such as delusions and hallucinations. However, they are less effective for other symptoms such as lack of motivation, poor memory, and problems with concentration.

>> **Antidepressant medications.** People with schizophrenia may have depression symptoms as well. Antidepressants are effective for treating these symptoms.

>> **Psychoeducation.** Psychoeducation means education and empowerment of the person and their family about their illness and how best to manage it. This helps to reduce relapse. Family tension, a common result of trying to deal with a poorly understood disability, may contribute to a relapse in the person with schizophrenia, and psychoeducation can help to avoid this.

>> **Cognitive behavioral therapy.** This type of psychological therapy can help reduce psychotic symptoms by helping the person to develop alternative explanations of schizophrenia symptoms, reducing the impact of the symptoms, and encouraging the person to take his or her medication.

>> **Social skills training.** This training is used to improve social and independent living skills.

>> **Assertive Community Treatment.** Assertive Community Treatment is an approach for people experiencing more severe illness. The care of the person is managed by a team of health professionals, such as psychiatrist, nurse, psychologist, and social worker. Care is available 24 hours a day and is tailored to the person's individual needs. Support is provided to family members as well. Assertive Community Treatment has been found to reduce relapse and the need for hospitalization.

BIPOLAR DISORDER TREATMENTS[84]

There is evidence that the following treatments help people with bipolar disorder:

>> **Medications.** A range of medications can help people with bipolar disorder. These include mood stabilizers, antipsychotics, and for some people, antidepressants.

>> **Psychoeducation.** Providing information to the person about bipolar disorder, its treatment, and managing its effect on his or her life. Psychoeducation has been found to reduce relapses when used together with medication.

>> **Psychological therapies.** Two therapies that research has found to be helpful are *cognitive behavioral therapy* and *interpersonal and social rhythm therapy.* CBT helps people monitor mood swings, overcome thinking patterns that affect mood, and function better. Interpersonal and social rhythm therapy covers potential problem areas in the person's life (grief, changes in roles, disputes, and interpersonal deficits) and helps them regulate social and sleep rhythms.

>> **Family therapy.** Educating family members on how they can support the person with bipolar disorder and avoid negative interactions that can trigger relapses has proven to be helpful for people with bipolar disorder.

A person who is experiencing severe psychosis may benefit from a short stay in the hospital to get back on track.

WHAT IF THE PERSON DOESN'T WANT HELP?

Some people may refuse to seek help even if they realize he or she is unwell. Their confusion and fear about what is happening to them may lead them to deny that anything is wrong. In this case, encourage them to talk to someone they trust. It is also possible that some may refuse to seek help because they lack insight that they are unwell. They might actively resist your attempts to encourage them to seek help. In either case, your course of action should depend on the type and severity of the person's symptoms.

It is important to recognize that unless a person with psychosis meets the criteria for involuntary committal procedures, they cannot be forced into treatment. If they are not at risk of harming themselves or others, remain patient, as people experiencing psychosis often need time to develop insight regarding their illness. Never threaten the person. Instead, remain friendly and open to the possibility that they may want your help in the future.

ACTION E: Encourage self-help and other support strategies

OTHER PEOPLE WHO CAN HELP

Try to determine whether the person has a supportive social network, and if they do, encourage them to utilize these supports.

Family, friends, and faith community networks are an important source of support for a person experiencing a disorder in which psychosis can occur.[32] A person is less likely to relapse if good relationships with family exist. [52, 116] Family and friends can help by

- Listening to the person without judging or being critical

- Keeping the person's life as stress-free as possible to reduce the chance of relapse

- Encouraging the person to get appropriate treatment and support

- Checking if the person is feeling suicidal and taking immediate action if the person is suicidal

- Providing the same support as they would for a physically ill person—including sending get-well cards, flowers, phoning or visiting the person, and helping out if they cannot manage

- Having an understanding of psychosis

- Looking for assistance from a support group

- Helping the person to develop an advance directive, wellness plan, relapse prevention plan, and/or personal directive.

Peer support and family support groups can be very helpful to the person experiencing psychosis and to family members.

SELF-HELP STRATEGIES

People experiencing psychosis should avoid the use of alcohol, marijuana, and other drugs. People sometimes take drugs as a way of coping with a developing psychotic illness, but these drugs can make the symptoms worse, initiate relapse, and make the disorder difficult to diagnose.[33] The use of marijuana can also slow recovery.[85]

Many people experiencing psychosis also have depression and/or an anxiety disorder. The self-help strategies recommended for depression and anxiety are also appropriate for people with psychosis. However, they should not to be used as the main form of assistance. Mental health professionals must be consulted.

What Is an Advance Directive?

An advance directive is a document describing how the person wants to be treated when they are unable to make their own decisions due to their present state of illness and appointing a person they trust to assist with the decision making at that time.

Helpful Resources

WEBSITES

Brain & Behavior Research Foundation

bbrfoundation.org/

This site provides downloadable fact sheets on psychotic disorders.

Mental Health America

www.mentalhealthamerica.net

Visit Mental Health America's site for information on mental health, getting help, and taking action.

National Alliance on Mental Illness

www.nami.org

NAMI is a nonprofit, grassroots, self-help, support and advocacy organization of individuals with mental disorders and their families. This website provides many resources on psychosis. The National Alliance on Mental Illness also offers peer support groups for families and consumers.

National Council for Behavioral Health

www.TheNationalCouncil.org

To locate mental health and addictions treatment facilities in your community, use the Find a Provider feature on the National Council's website.

National Institute of Mental Health

www.nimh.nih.gov

This U.S. government site gives a wealth of up-to-date information on psychosis in the form of downloadable booklets and fact sheets.

Pendulum

www.pendulum.org

Pendulum is a nonprofit organization providing information on bipolar disorder. The website includes book reviews, discussion forums, articles, and links to other resources.

Schizophrenia.com

www.schizophrenia.com

This website provides information, support, and education to family members, caregivers, and individuals whose lives have been affected by schizophrenia.

BOOKS

Bauer, M. S., Kilbourne, A. M., Greenwald, D. E. and Ludman, E. (2009) *Overcoming bipolar disorder.* New Harbinger Publications, Oakland, CA.
A self-help guide for people in treatment for bipolar disorder. Includes strategies for preventing relapse, safe and effective goal setting, and medication.

Mondimore, F. M. (2006) *Bipolar disorder: a guide for patients and families* (revised edition). Johns Hopkins University Press, Baltimore, MD.
This book has won a number of awards for contributing to the public's awareness and better understanding of mental illness.

Temes, R. (2002) *Getting your life back together when you have schizophrenia.* New Harbinger Publications, Oakland, CA.
This is a self-help guide for people starting a treatment program for schizophrenia. It includes information about what to expect from medication and therapy and strategies for improving overall quality of life.

HELP LINES

American Psychiatric Association Answer Center

1-888-35-PSYCH (1-888-357-7924)
Live operators from 8:30 a.m. to 6 p.m., Eastern time, refer you to local board-certified psychiatrist.

SUPPORT GROUPS

National Alliance on Mental Illness

www.nami.org

On the home page, click on "Find Support."

Recovery International

www.recovery-inc.com

On the home page, click on "Find a Meeting"
to find the next Recovery International meeting
in your area.

Recovery International, a Chicago-based
self-help mental health organization,
sponsors weekly group peer-led meetings
in many communities, as well as telephone
and Internet-based meetings.

Schizophrenia and Related Disorders Alliance of America

www.sardaa.org/schizophrenics-anonymous/

Schizophrenics Anonymous is comprised
of self-help groups established to support
the recovery of people who experience
schizophrenia. The website lists location
of self-help groups.

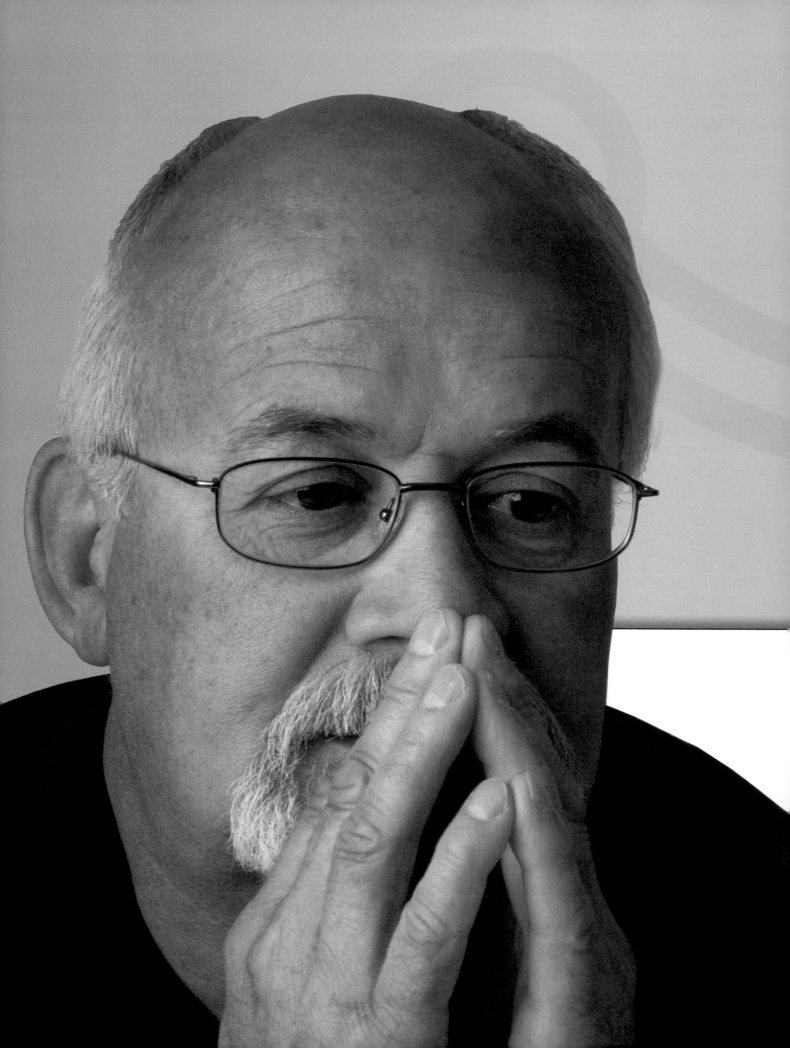

CHAPTER 6

Substance Use Disorders

What Is a Substance Use Disorder?

Different substances affect the brain in different ways. People use substances because of these effects, which include increasing feelings of pleasure or decreasing feelings of distress. Using alcohol and/or other drugs does not in itself mean that a person has a substance use disorder.

Substance use disorders include any of the following:[21]

- *Abuse* of alcohol or other drugs which leads to work, school, home, health, or legal problems

- *Dependence* on alcohol or other drugs.

The symptoms of substance dependence are

- Tolerance for the substance (the person needs increased amounts over time or gets less effect with repeated use)

- Problems with withdrawal (the person experiences withdrawal symptoms or uses substance to relieve withdrawal symptoms)

- Use of larger amounts over longer periods than intended

- Problems in cutting down or controlling use

- A lot of time spent getting the substance, using it, or recovering from its effects

- The person gives up or reduces important social, occupational, or recreational activities because of substance use

- The person continues using the substance despite knowing that use has negative consequences.

Approximately 8 percent of U.S. adults have a substance use disorder[90] in a given year, with the majority involving alcohol. Substance use disorders tend to begin in adolescence or early adulthood with a median age of onset of 20 years[2] (half the people have developed the disorder by this age), and 75 percent develop substance use disorder by age 27. Substance use disorders are more than twice as common in males as in females. Substance use disorders often co-occur with mood, anxiety, and psychotic disorders. People with a mood or anxiety disorder are two to three times more likely to have a substance use disorder.[86] One reason for this is that many people use alcohol or other drugs as self-medication for anxiety, depression, or psychosis.

Alcohol

Alcohol makes people less alert and impairs concentration and coordination. Some people use alcohol to reduce anxiety, and in the short term, it can help. In small quantities, alcohol causes people to relax and lower their inhibitions. They can feel more confident and often act more extroverted. However, alcohol use can produce a range of short-term and long-term problems.

Short-Term Problems Caused by Alcohol Intoxication

When a person is intoxicated, they are at risk for a number of problems, such as

>> **Physical injuries.** People are more likely to engage in risky behavior, which can lead to injury or death. Alcohol is a big contributor to traffic accidents. Also, intoxication can lead to poor motor coordination, resulting

in staggering or falling, slurred speech, and even medical emergencies such as continual vomiting or unconsciousness.

>> **Aggression and antisocial behavior.** People can become aggressive and are at a higher risk of committing crimes.

>> **Sexual risk taking.** Risks include not using condoms or contraceptives and having multiple sexual partners. The consequences of these behaviors can be unwanted sexual contact, unwanted pregnancy, and sexually transmitted diseases.

>> **Suicide and self-injury.** When a person is intoxicated, they are prone to suicide or self-injury. Alcohol increases risk in several ways. It can

- Intensify feelings of anxiety, depression, and anger

- Inhibit the use of effective coping strategies

- Make a person more likely to act on suicidal feelings.

Long-Term Problems Caused by Alcohol Use

With heavy and prolonged use, alcohol can cause problems in many areas—physical, psychological, and social:

>> **Alcohol use disorders.** People who regularly drink alcohol above recommended levels, particularly those who start at an early age, have an increased risk of developing an alcohol use disorder.

>> **Other substance use disorders.** People who use alcohol are more likely to be introduced to other drugs.

>> **Depression and anxiety.** People who suffer from anxiety or depressive disorders and drink heavily can show rapid improvement in their mood when they cut out alcohol.[61] If a person is feeling suicidal,

they are more likely to attempt suicide when under the influence of alcohol.

>> **Social problems.** Abuse of alcohol is associated with family conflict, dropping out of school, unemployment, and social isolation.

>> **Physical health problems.** In the long term, heavy alcohol use can produce problems such as liver disease, brain damage, heart impairment, muscle weakness, pancreatitis, ulcers and gastrointestinal bleeding, nerve damage to hands and feet, and weight gain.

How Much Is Too Much?

Many people consume alcohol, and in most cases this will not damage their health. The U.S. government has defined the risk of alcohol consumption as follows:[87]

Low-risk drinking:

> **Men:** two drinks per day
> **Women:** one drink per day

Because of age-related changes in the body, people older than 65 are recommended to consume no more than one drink per day.

At-risk or problem drinking:

> **Men:** more than four drinks per occasion or more than 14 per week
> **Women:** more than three drinks per occasion or more than seven per week

Because drinks vary in size and amount of alcohol they contain, a standard drink has been defined as one that contains 14 grams of pure alcohol—see examples in the box on the next page.

U.S. Standard Drink Equivalents[88]

Each of the following is equivalent to one standard drink:*

- 12 oz. beer (approx. 5% alcohol content)

- 8–9 oz. malt liquor (approx. 7% alcohol content)

- 5 oz. table wine (approx. 12% alcohol content)

- 3–4 oz. fortified wine such as sherry or port (approx. 17% alcohol content)

- 2–3 oz. cordial, liqueur, or aperitif (approx. 24% alcohol content)

- 1.5 oz. brandy (a single jigger) (approx. 40% alcohol content)

- 1.5 oz. spirits, such as a single jigger of 80-proof gin, vodka, whiskey (approx. 40% alcohol content).

*THESE ARE APPROXIMATE, SINCE DIFFERENT BRANDS AND TYPES OF BEVERAGES VARY IN ACTUAL ALCOHOL CONTENT

People who drink above these alcohol recommendations are at risk of developing physical and mental health problems. The RAPS4 Questionnaire was developed as a brief screening device to assess whether people have an alcohol use disorder.[89] The RAPS4 gets its name from the questions it poses to the person, which pertain to remorse (R), amnesia (A), performance (P), and starter drinking behavior (S).

The Rapid Alcohol Problems Screen (RAPS4)[89]

>> During the past year, have you had a feeling of guilt or remorse after drinking?

>> During the past year, has a friend or family member ever told you about things you said or did while you were drinking that you could not remember?

>> During the past year, have you failed to do what was normally expected from you because of drinking?

>> Do you sometimes take a drink in the morning when you first get up?

NOTE: A "YES" ANSWER TO AT LEAST ONE OF THE FOUR QUESTIONS SUGGESTS THAT A PERSON'S DRINKING IS HARMFUL TO THEIR HEALTH AND WELL-BEING AND MAY ADVERSELY AFFECT THEIR WORK AND THOSE AROUND THEM. IN THIS CASE, THE PERSON SHOULD GET A FULL EVALUATION FROM A QUALIFIED PROFESSIONAL.

Other Drugs

The diagram below shows the relative occurrence of various drug use disorders in the United States.[90]

PAST YEAR DEPENDENCE OR ABUSE, 2011

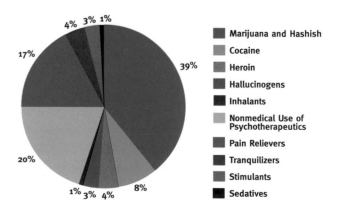

- Marijuana and Hashish
- Cocaine
- Heroin
- Hallucinogens
- Inhalants
- Nonmedical Use of Psychotherapeutics
- Pain Relievers
- Tranquilizers
- Stimulants
- Sedatives

Marijuana (Cannabis)

Marijuana is a mind-altering drug and is a mixture of dried, shredded leaves, stems, seeds, and flowers of the hemp plant. Marijuana, or cannabis has street names such as *pot, herb, weed, grass, boom, Mary Jane, gangster, or chronic.*

The main active chemical in marijuana is THC (delta-9-tetrahydrocannabinol). Marijuana's effects on the user vary depending on how much THC it contains. The THC content of marijuana has been increasing since the 1970s. Use of marijuana can interfere with performance at work or school and lead to increased risk of accidents if used while driving or operating machinery. The 2011 National Survey on Drug Use and Health showed that 7 percent of people aged 12 or older used marijuana in the past month.[90] Although it is the most commonly used illicit drug in the United States, most users do not develop a substance use disorder.

Marijuana abuse is associated with other mental health problems. People who use marijuana are more likely to suffer from a range of other mental health problems, including anxiety and depression, but it is unclear which comes first. Also, marijuana use by adolescents and young adults has been found to increase the risk of developing schizophrenia, particularly in persons with a personal or family history of schizophrenia.[68]

Opioid Drugs (Including Heroin)

Opioid drugs include heroin, morphine, opium, and codeine. Heroin is processed from morphine, which is a naturally occurring substance taken from the Asian poppy plant. Street names for heroin include *smack, H, skag,* and *junk.* Although heroin gets lots of publicity, it is not a widely used drug in the United States. In 2011, it was estimated that 0.2 percent of Americans used heroin.[90] However, it is a highly addictive drug, and most people who use it develop a substance use disorder. Heroin produces a short-term feeling of euphoria, well-being, and relief of pain. Most people who are dependent on heroin have associated problems such as depression, alcohol dependence, and criminal behavior. People who use heroin are at higher risk for suicide.

Sedatives and Tranquilizers

These are prescription drugs used to treat anxiety and sleep problems. However, some people use them for nonmedical purposes. A 2011 national survey showed that 2.4 percent of people aged 12 or older used these types of prescription drugs for nonmedical purposes in the past month.[90] Abuse of these drugs can lead to dangerous situations, such as driving while under the influence.

Even when used under prescription, some people become dependent on these medications after long-term use. Older people are the most likely to be affected. When used long-term, these medications can increase the risk of falls and cognitive impairment in older people.

Cocaine

Cocaine is a highly addictive stimulant drug. Cocaine is generally sold on the street in the form of a white powder known as *coke, C, snowflake,* or *blow.* Although sometimes thought of as a modern drug problem, cocaine has been abused for more than a century, and the coca leaves from which it is made have been used for thousands of years. A 2011 national survey showed that 0.5 percent of people aged 12 or older used cocaine in the past month.[90] Cocaine gives very strong euphoric effects, and people can develop dependence after using it for a very short time. With long-term use, people can develop mental health problems such as paranoia, aggression, anxiety, and depression.

Amphetamines (Including Methamphetamine and Dextroamphetamine)

Amphetamines belong to a category of stimulant drugs and have the temporary effect of increasing energy and apparent mental alertness. However, as the effect wears off, a person may experience a range of problems including depression, irritability, agitation, craving, increased appetite, and sleepiness. Amphetamines come in many shapes and forms and are taken in many ways. They can be in the form of powder, tablets, capsules, crystals, or liquid.

Methamphetamine has a chemical structure similar to amphetamine but has a stronger effect on the brain. The effects of methamphetamine can last 6 to 8 hours. After the initial "rush," there is a state of agitation, which in some individuals can lead to violent behavior. Common names for methamphetamine are *speed, meth,* or *chalk.* In its smoked form, it can be referred to as *ice, crystal, crank,* or *glass.*

High doses of amphetamine can lead to aggression, intense anxiety, paranoia, and psychotic symptoms. Withdrawal symptoms can include temporary depression. A particular mental health risk is amphetamine psychosis or "speed" psychosis, which involves symptoms similar to schizophrenia. The person may experience hallucinations, delusions, and uncontrolled violent behavior. The person will recover as the drug wears off but is vulnerable to further episodes of drug-induced psychosis if the drug is used again.

Some types of amphetamines have legitimate medical uses. They are used under prescription to treat attention-deficit/hyperactivity disorder and some other medical conditions.

Hallucinogens (Including Ecstasy)

Hallucinogens are drugs that affect a person's perceptions of reality. Some hallucinogens also produce rapid, intense emotional changes. In a 2011 survey, it was found that 0.4 percent of people aged 12 or older used hallucinogens in the past month.[90] The most widely used hallucinogenic drug is LSD. A particular problem associated with hallucinogens is flashbacks, where the person reexperiences some perceptual effects of the drug when they have not been recently using it.

Ecstasy (MDMA also known as "E") is a stimulant drug with hallucinogenic properties. Use of this drug has been rising steadily since the early 1990s. Some young people use it as a "party drug" and at social gatherings called "raves." Users can develop an adverse reaction that in extreme cases can lead to death. To reduce this risk, users need to maintain a steady fluid intake and rest. While intoxicated, ecstasy users report that they feel emotionally close to others. When coming off the drug, they often experience depressed mood. The long-term effects of using ecstasy are of particular concern. There is considerable evidence that ecstasy damages nerve cells in the brain that use a chemical messenger called *serotonin.*[92] Research on people who have used ecstasy regularly shows that they have reduced sexual interest and a range of mental health problems.

Inhalants

Inhalants are breathable chemical vapors that produce mind-altering effects. The effects of inhalants range from an alcohol-like intoxication and euphoria to hallucinations, depending on the substance and the dosage. These include solvents (paint thinners, gasoline, glues), gases (aerosols, butane lighters), and nitrites.

Although people are exposed to volatile solvents and other inhalants in the home and workplace, many do not think of inhalable substances as drugs. Young people are the most likely to abuse inhalants, partly because inhalants are readily available and inexpensive. In 2011, approximately 0.2 percent of people aged 12 or older used inhalants in the past month.[90]

The intentional misuse of common household products to get high can be fatal. Some people suffer "sudden sniffing death syndrome," while others become addicted. Young people are usually unaware of the serious health risks, and those who start using them at an early age are likely to become dependent on them. These agents destroy cells in the brain, the liver, and the kidneys.

Tobacco

A 2011 survey found that tobacco was used by 26.5 percent of people aged 12 or older in the past month.[90] Tobacco is so widely used that we do not usually think of it as a mental health issue. However, there is a high rate of mental health problems in people who use tobacco. People with mental disorders are nearly twice as likely to smoke cigarettes as people without.[93] Use is particularly high in people with schizophrenia (70-90 percent in people with long-term schizophrenia).[94] It is possible that some people with mental disorders use tobacco as a type of self-medication in order to improve mood and cognitive functioning.

What Causes Substance Use Disorders?

Most of our knowledge about the causes of substance use disorders relates to alcohol, but the causes of other drug use disorders are likely to be similar.

There is no single cause of alcohol use disorders. Many factors increase a person's chances of developing such a disorder,[34] including

>> **Availability and tolerance of alcohol in society.** Where alcohol is readily available and socially acceptable, alcohol use disorders are more likely to develop. This applies not only to society as a whole, but also to particular social groups.

>> **Social factors.** Certain groups are prone to alcohol use disorders, including males, people with low education and income, people who have divorced, and people in certain occupations with a drinking culture.

>> **Genetic predisposition.** People who have a biological parent with an alcohol use disorder are more likely to develop the disorder, even if adopted into a family with no alcohol use disorder.

>> **Alcohol sensitivity.** Some people are physiologically less sensitive to the effects of alcohol than others, and these people are more likely to drink heavily and develop an alcohol use disorder.

>> **Learning.** People can learn a habit of heavy drinking. This habit is maintained because alcohol has been associated with pleasant effects or a reduction of stress.

>> **Other mental health problems.** People who have other mental disorders may use alcohol as a type of self-medication.

Importance of Early Intervention for Substance Use Disorders

It is easier for someone to recover from a substance use problem if detected and treated early, rather than after they become dependent on the substance. Early intervention will prevent many of the long-term ill effects on a person's physical health, social relationships, educational progress, financial status, and job prospects. It will also reduce the possibility of serious problems with the law. Substance use problems typically begin in adolescence and early adulthood, so this is the critical time for early intervention.

The Mental Health First Aid Action Plan for Substance Use Disorders

MENTAL HEALTH FIRST AID ACTION PLAN	
ACTION A	Assess for risk of suicide or harm
ACTION L	Listen nonjudgmentally
ACTION G	Give reassurance and information
ACTION E	Encourage appropriate professional help
ACTION E®	Encourage self-help and other support strategies

Alcohol use disorders are the major type of substance use disorders in the United States.[1] In this section, the MHFA® Action Plan is applied to problem drinking but can be generalized to help people with problems with other drugs.

ACTION A: Assess for risk of suicide or harm[95]

If you are concerned about someone's drinking, talk to the person about it openly and honestly. Talk with them in a quiet, private environment at a time when there will be no interruptions and when both of you are sober and are in a calm frame of mind. Consider the following as part of the assessment approach:

>> **Perception of their drinking.** Try to understand the person's own perception of their drinking. Ask about their drinking behavior (for example, about how much alcohol the person tends to drink) and if they believe their drinking is a problem.

>> **Readiness to talk.** Consider the person's readiness to talk about his or her drinking problem by asking about areas of life that it may be affecting, such as mood, work performance, and relationships. The person may deny, or might not recognize, he or she has a drinking problem. Trying to force the person to admit a problem may cause conflict.

>> **Use "I" statements.** Express your point of view by using "I" statements—for example, "I am concerned about how much you've been drinking lately." Identify and discuss the person's behavior rather than criticize their character—for example, "Your drinking seems to be getting in the way of your friendships," rather than "You're a pathetic drunk."

>> Recall of events. When discussing the person's drinking, keep in mind the person may recall events that occurred while they were drinking in a different way than how they actually happened, or they may not recall events at all.

There are four main crises that may be associated with problem drinking:

1. The person is *intoxicated, has alcohol poisoning, or is in severe withdrawal.*

2. The person is *aggressive.*

3. The person has *suicidal thoughts and behaviors.*

4. The person is engaging in *nonsuicidal self-injury.*

The first crises (*intoxication, alcohol poisoning, severe withdrawal,* and *aggression*) will be observed more in the behavior of the person than what they tell you, whereas the last crises (*suicidal thoughts and behaviors* and *nonsuicidal self-injury*) will only become apparent after you have approached the person about your concerns. A person who is depressed and also has an alcohol problem has a much higher risk of suicide and self-injury. Of the people who complete suicide, 26 percent had a substance use disorder.[44]

For more information on warning signs of suicide, see Action A in Chapter 3.

If the person is using alcohol heavily, it is possible they will experience a medical emergency from alcohol intoxication, alcohol poisoning, or withdrawal symptoms.

ALCOHOL INTOXICATION AND POISONING MAY LEAD TO A MEDICAL EMERGENCY

Call an ambulance, or seek medical help, *in any of the following circumstances:*

- Continual vomiting

- Vomiting while unconscious

- The person cannot be awakened or falls into an unconscious state

- Signs of a possible head injury, such as vomiting and talking incoherently

- Drink spiking is suspected

- Irregular, shallow, or slow breathing

- Irregular, weak, or slow pulse rate

- Cold, clammy, pale, or bluish skin.

SEVERE ALCOHOL WITHDRAWAL MAY LEAD TO A MEDICAL EMERGENCY

Seek medical help if the person displays symptoms of severe alcohol withdrawal, such as

- Delirium tremens (a state of confusion and visual hallucinations)

- Agitation

- Fever

- Seizures

- Blackout—when the person forgets what happened during the drinking episode.

If you have no concerns the person is in crisis, move on to another Action.

Let the person know that you are concerned and are willing to help.

- If there is concern that the person is **intoxicated, poisoned, or in a state of withdrawal**, see *First Aid for a Medical Emergency from Alcohol Abuse*.

- If there is concern that the person is **aggressive**, see *First Aid for Aggressive Behavior*.

- If there is concern about **suicidal thoughts**, see *First Aid for Suicidal Thoughts and Behaviors*.

  If you have serious concerns, call 911 or the National Suicide Prevention Lifeline at 1-800-273-TALK (8255).

- If there is concern about **nonsuicidal self-injury**, see *First Aid for Nonsuicidal Self-Injury*.

ACTION L: Listen nonjudgmentally

This conversation might be the first time the person has thought about their drinking as a problem.

- Listen without judging the person as bad or immoral.

- Avoid expressing moral judgments about their drinking.

- Do not be critical. You are more likely to be able to help them in the long term if you maintain a noncritical but concerned approach.

- Do not label the person or accuse the person of being an alcoholic.

- Try not to express your frustration at the person for having alcohol use problems.

See Action L in Chapter 3 for more tips on nonjudgmental listening.

ACTION G: Give reassurance and information

TREAT THE PERSON WITH RESPECT AND DIGNITY
Interact with the person in a supportive way rather than threatening, confronting, or lecturing the person.

HAVE REALISTIC EXPECTATIONS FOR THE PERSON
Do not expect a change in the person's thinking or behavior right away. Major behavior changes take time to be achieved and often involve the person going through a number of stages (see box on *The Stages of Change*). Keep in mind that

- Changing drinking habits is not easy.

- Willpower and self-resolve are not always enough to stop problem drinking.

- Advice alone may not help the person change their drinking behavior.

- If abstinence from drinking is not the person's goal, reducing the quantity of alcohol consumed is still a worthwhile objective.

- A person may attempt to change or stop drinking more than once before they are successful.

The Stages of Change[96]

People who have a substance use disorder may not want to change. The person could be in any of the following stages:

1. *Precontemplation*. The person sees no need to change.

2. *Contemplation*. The person has thought of the pros and cons of their substance use but is not sure about changing.

3. *Preparation*. The person is ready to take action to change.

4. *Action*. The person is attempting to change and avoiding situations that might trigger substance use.

5. *Maintenance*. The person has changed and is working to prevent a relapse.

6. *Relapse*. The person may relapse once or several times before changing their drinking patterns.

SUPPORTING THE PERSON WHO DOES NOT WANT TO CHANGE

If the person is unwilling to change their drinking behavior, you can speak with a health professional to determine how best to approach the person about your concerns, or you could consult with others who have dealt with problem drinking about effective ways to help. You could discuss with the person the link between drinking behavior and the negative consequences.

If the person is unwilling to change their drinking behavior, do not

- Join in drinking with the person

- Try to control the person by bribing, nagging, threatening, or crying

- Make excuses for the person or cover up their drinking or behavior

- Take on the person's responsibilities, except if not doing so would cause harm to their own life or others

- Feel guilty or responsible.

SUPPORTING THE PERSON WHO DOES WANT TO CHANGE

Tell the person what you are willing and able to do to help. This may range from simply being a good listener to organizing professional help.

Encouraging low-risk drinking. To encourage low-risk drinking, the following may assist the person to change his or her drinking behaviors:

- Help them to realize that only they can take responsibility for reducing their alcohol intake and that although changing drinking patterns is difficult, they should not give up trying.

- Encourage and assist the person to find some information on how to reduce the harms associated with problem drinking.

- If appropriate, inform the person that alcohol may interact with other drugs (illicit or prescribed) in an unpredictable way, which may lead to a medical emergency.

- Ask the person if he or she would like some tips on low-risk drinking (see box).

Practical Tips for Low-Risk Drinking

>> Know what a standard drink is and the number of standard drinks they consume

>> Know the alcohol content of their drink

>> See if the number of standard drinks is listed on the beverage's packaging

>> Eat while drinking

>> Drink plenty of water on a drinking occasion to prevent dehydration

>> Drink beverages with lower alcohol content (e.g., light beer instead of full-strength beer)

>> Switch to nonalcoholic drinks when they start to feel the effects of alcohol

>> Do not let others top up their drink before it is finished, so as not to lose track of how much alcohol they have consumed

>> Avoid keeping up with their friends drink for drink

>> Avoid participating in drinking competitions and drinking games

>> Drink slowly, for example, by taking sips instead of gulps and putting the drink down between sips

>> Have one drink at a time

>> Spend their time in activities that don't involve drinking

>> Make drinking alcohol a complementary activity instead of the sole activity

>> Identify situations where drinking is likely and avoid them, if practical.

Managing social pressure to drink. There is often social pressure to get drunk when drinking. Encourage the person to be assertive when they feel pressured to drink more than they intend. Tell the person that they have the right to refuse alcohol. Tell them that they can say "no thanks" without explanation, or suggest different ways they can say "no," such as "I don't feel like it," "I don't feel well," or "I am taking medication." Encourage the person to practice different ways of saying "no." Suggest to the person that saying "no" to alcohol gets easier the more they do it and that the people who care about them will accept their decision not to drink or to reduce the amount that they drink.

ACTION E: Encourage appropriate professional help

Many people with alcohol and drug problems do not receive any treatment for these problems. In the United States, only 38 percent of people with a substance use disorder in the past year received such help.[30] Even when people do seek help, they can delay for many years. Delays of 5 to 10 years are not unusual.[31] These delays can cause problems for family life and occupation, damage their physical health, and increase the risk for other mental disorders such as depression and anxiety.

DISCUSS OPTIONS FOR SEEKING PROFESSIONAL HELP

Tell the person that you will support them in getting professional help. If the person is willing to seek professional help, give them information about local options and encourage them to make an appointment.

PROFESSIONALS WHO CAN HELP

A variety of health professionals can provide help to a person with alcohol problems. They are

- Primary care physicians

- Drug and alcohol specialists

- Mental health professionals

- Certified peer specialists.

More information about how these professionals can help is available in Chapter 1.

If the person is uncertain about what to do, encourage the person to consult a primary care physician first. People are more likely to reduce their substance use if the primary care physician

- Tests the person to see if the alcohol or other substances have caused harm to the body

- Gives information on the harms involved

- Gives clear advice to cut down or stop substance use.

>> **Drug and alcohol specialists.** A person with an alcohol or other drug problem may be helped by a certified substance abuse treatment counselor or a certified substance abuse treatment program. Always look for credentials that demonstrate a professional has specific training and competence in treating people with substance use disorders. Professional substance abuse treatment can be offered on an inpatient, outpatient, or residential basis, depending upon the severity of illness.

>> **Mental health professionals.** The person may be drinking as a means of coping with other problems, such as underlying emotional distress or an untreated mental disorder. Furthermore, mental health problems can be caused or exacerbated by drinking alcohol. Usually, to stop problem drinking, the person's underlying emotional distress or mental health problems will need to be addressed. In this case, the most appropriate professional may be a psychologist or a psychiatrist.

TREATMENTS AVAILABLE FOR ALCOHOL PROBLEMS

The treatments for problem alcohol use depend on severity, how motivated the person is to change, and what other physical and mental health problems they also have. The following treatments are known to be effective:[97]

>> **Brief intervention.** If a person is drinking at a level that could damage their health, then brief counseling by a health care professional can help them reduce or stop drinking. If they have an alcohol use disorder, it can help to motivate them to enter long-term treatment. This type of intervention generally takes four or fewer sessions, each lasting from a few minutes up to an hour. The health care professional looks at how much the person is drinking, gives information about risks to their health, advises them to cut down, discusses options for how to change, motivates the person to act by emphasizing personal responsibility, and monitors progress. In doing these things, the health care professional adopts an empathic rather than a coercive approach.

>> **Alcohol use disorder treatment.** If the person has an alcohol use disorder, then treatment needs to do several things:

- Overcome any physiological dependence on alcohol

- Overcome any psychological dependence, such as using alcohol to help the person cope with anxiety or depression

- Overcome habits that have been formed, such as a social life that revolves around drinking.

>> **Withdrawal management.** If the person is dependent on alcohol, they will have to withdraw from alcohol before other approaches are tried. This should be done under professional supervision. However, withdrawal is not enough and should be combined with other treatments to prevent the person from relapsing. It is only part of the recovery process, and many lifestyle changes are required to change drinking behaviors.

>> **Psychological treatments.** These include

- Cognitive behavioral therapy (which teaches the person how to cope with cravings and how to recognize and cope with situations that might trigger relapse)

- Motivational enhancement therapy (which helps motivate and empower a person to change)

>> **Medications.** There are a number of types of medications that can assist a person to stay off alcohol. These include anticraving medications (such as naltrexone), medications that give an unpleasant effect if the person drinks (disulfiram, also known as Antabuse), or medications for the treatment of underlying anxiety and depression.

WHAT IF THE PERSON DOESN'T WANT HELP?

The person may not want professional help when it is first suggested and may find it difficult to accept. If this is the case, explain to the person that there are several approaches available for treating drinking problems. If the person won't seek help because he or she doesn't want to stop drinking completely, explain the treatment goal may be to reduce alcohol consumption rather than to quit altogether. Reassure the person that professional help is confidential.

If the person is unwilling to seek professional help, you should set boundaries around what behavior you are willing and not willing to accept from the person. It is important to continue to suggest professional help if the person is putting himself or herself or others at risk of harm.

Be prepared to talk to the person about seeking professional help again in the future. Be compassionate and patient while waiting for the person to accept their need for professional help—it is ultimately the person's decision. Remember the person cannot be forced to get professional help except under certain circumstances—for example, if a violent incident results in law enforcement being called or following a medical emergency.

ACTION E: Encourage self-help and other support strategies

ROLE OF FAMILY AND FRIENDS IN RECOVERY

Research has shown that people are more likely to recover if they have[98]

- Stable family relationships

- Approval and sympathy expressed by their families

- Supportive friends

- Friends who don't use alcohol or other drugs and encourage the person not to use.

Family and friends can play an important role in the recovery of a person with an alcohol or other drug problem. Encourage them to reach out to friends and family who support their efforts to change their drinking behaviors and to spend time with supportive nondrinking friends or family. Family and friends can help the person to seek treatment and support to change their drinking behavior. They can also help reduce the chances of a relapse after a person has stopped substance use. People are more likely to start using again if there is an emotional upset in their life, and family and friends can try to reduce this possibility. It is useful to warn the person that not all family and friends will be supportive of his or her efforts.

There are numerous groups that support individuals recovering from substance use by providing mutual support and information. Twelve-step programs, such as Alcoholics Anonymus (AA) and Narcotics Anonymus (NA), are self-help groups in which people work to follow steps to recovery. There are also support groups for families of the substance user such as AL-ANON, Alateen, Adult Children of Alcoholics, Nar-ANON, Rational Recovery, and Celebrate Recovery.

Helpful Resources

FOR SUBSTANCE USE DISORDERS

WEBSITES

Centers for Disease Control and Prevention
www.smokefree.gov
Smokefree.gov, created by the Centers for Disease Control and Prevention, provides ideas about how to stop using tobacco. Includes downloadable resources and contacts for online and phone counseling.

Mental Health America
www.mentalhealthamerica.net
Visit Mental Health America's site for information on mental health, getting help, and taking action.

National Council for Behavioral Health
www.TheNationalCouncil.org
To locate mental health and addictions treatment facilities in your community, use the Find a Provider feature on the National Council's website.

National Council on Alcoholism and Drug Dependence, Inc.
www.ncadd.org
This site features information on local resources for getting help for a substance use concern, fact sheets, and further information for friends, family members, parents, and youth on having a conversation about substance use.

National Institute on Alcohol Abuse And Alcoholism
www.niaaa.nih.gov
The National Institute on Alcohol Abuse and Alcoholism is the lead agency for U.S. research on alcohol use disorders and health.

National Institute on Drug Abuse

www.nida.nih.gov

Provides links to information for parents, teens, health professionals, teachers, and others about drugs of all types.

Substance Abuse and Mental Health Services Administration

www.samhsa.gov

www.findtreatment.samhsa.gov/

The Substance Abuse and Mental Health Services Administration (SAMHSA) website has information about substance use disorders of all kinds. It has information for the public, including families, health professionals, schools, and individuals. It also includes a treatment finder to locate a substance use treatment provider in your area.

SCREENING SITES

Do I have a drug problem?

www.drugscreening.org

How much is too much?

www.alcoholscreening.org

These websites were developed by the Boston University School of Public Health. They provide online tests about your own, or someone else's, level of drug use, including advice about cutting down or getting professional treatment.

BOOKS

Fanning, P. (1996) *The addiction workbook.* New Harbinger Publications, Oakland, CA. This self-help guide may assist some people to overcome their alcohol or other drug dependence disorder.

Olsen, P. and Levounis, P. (2008) *Sober siblings: how to help your alcoholic brother or sister—and not lose yourself.* Da Capo Press, Cambridge, MA. This book was written by the sober sister of two brothers with alcohol dependence and a drug and alcohol rehabilitation professional. It includes personal recollections as well as practical advice for helping a sibling recover from alcohol abuse.

Rotgers, F. (2002) *Responsible drinking: a moderation management approach for problem drinkers with worksheet.* New Harbinger Publications, Oakland, CA. This book may assist people who are not addicted to alcohol, but wish to curb their use, to determine their own ideal drinking levels and stick to them.

The Healing Project (2008) *Voices of alcoholism.* LaChance Publishing, Brooklyn, NY. True stories of recovery from alcohol dependence.

HELP LINES FOR TOBACCO CESSATION

National Cancer Institute Smoking Quitline

1-877-44U-QUIT (1-877-448-7848)
(English and Spanish)

Smoking Cessation Centers

1-800-QUIT-NOW (1-800-784-8669)
(number used in 17 states; English
and Spanish)

SUPPORT GROUPS

Al-Anon and Alateen

www.al-anon.org
www.alateen.org
Provides information and support for the family
members and friends of people with alcohol
problems. Includes a list of meetings in the United
States and Canada.

American Self-Help Group Clearinghouse

www.mentalhelp.net/selfhelp/
This searchable database of more than 1,100 self-help
and caregiver support groups includes many for
addictions and other substance use disorders. Also
listed are local self-help clearinghouses worldwide,
research studies, information on starting face-to-face
and online groups, and a registry for persons interested
in starting national or international self-help groups.

Narcotics Anonymous and Alcoholics Anonymous

www.na.org
www.aa.org
These websites will give you information on Narcotics
Anonymous and Alcoholics Anonymous and will give
you the website and contacts for groups in your area.

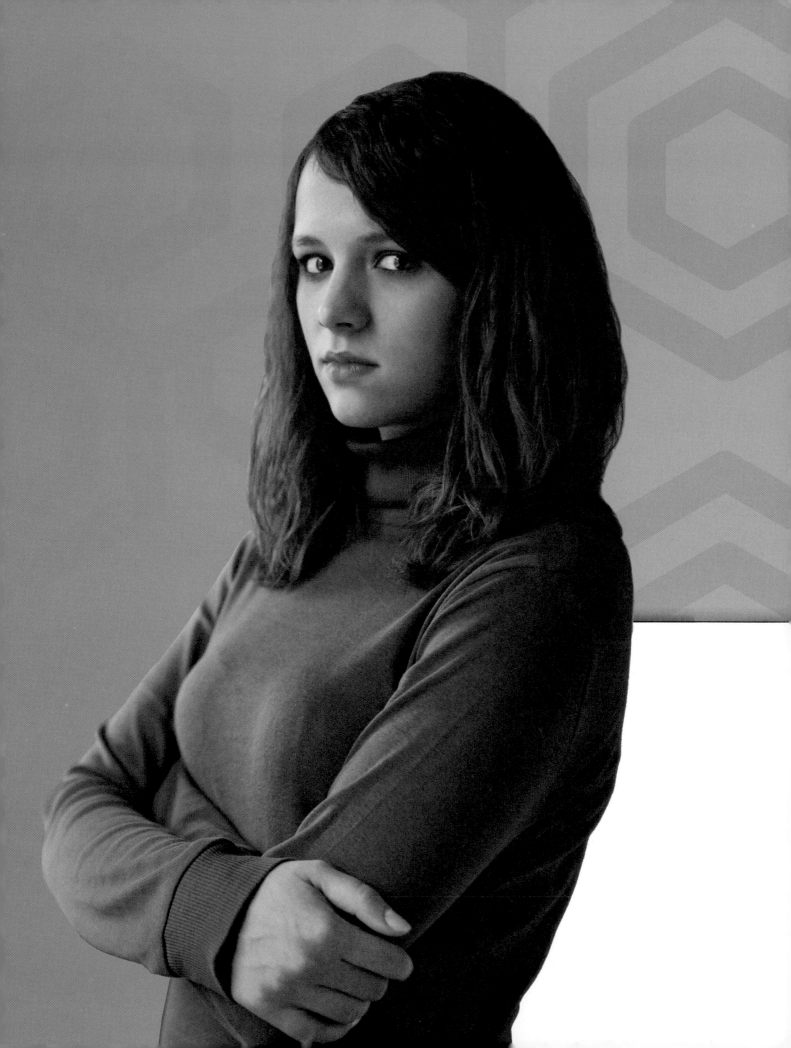

CHAPTER 7

Eating Disorders

What Are Eating Disorders?

A person with an eating disorder can be underweight, normal weight, or overweight. Most individuals with eating disorders are very distressed with concerns of appearing overweight and/or physically unattractive. Eating disorders are not just about food, weight, vanity, or willpower, but are serious and potentially life-threatening mental disorders. Most eating disorders occur when a person has distortions in thoughts and emotions relating to body image, leading to marked changes in eating or exercise behaviors that interfere with the person's life.

Eating disorders are two to three times more common in females than in males.[99] The median age of onset for eating disorders ranges from 18 to 20 years (50 percent have onset before these ages). A high proportion of people with eating disorders also have another mental disorder, particularly anxiety, mood, or substance use disorders. However, less than a third of people with eating disorders had received treatment for a mental health problem in the past 12 months.

Warning Signs an Eating Disorder Is Developing

It is important to know the warning signs that an eating disorder is developing. These include behavioral, physical, and psychological signs.[100]

BEHAVIORAL WARNING SIGNS

- Dieting behaviors, such as fasting, counting calories, avoidance of food groups or types

- Evidence of binge eating (disappearance or hoarding of food)

- Evidence of vomiting or laxative use (making trips to the bathroom during or immediately after meals)

- Excessive, obsessive, or ritualistic exercise patterns (exercising when injured or in bad weather, feeling compelled to perform a certain number of repetitions of exercises, or experiencing distress if unable to exercise)

- Changes in food preferences (refusing to eat certain fatty or bad foods, cutting out whole food groups such as meat or dairy, claiming to dislike foods previously enjoyed, developing a sudden concern with healthy eating, or replacing meals with fluids)

- Development of rigid patterns around food selection, preparation, and eating, such as cutting food into small pieces, or eating very slowly

- Avoidance of eating meals, especially when in a social setting (skipping meals by claiming they have already eaten or have an intolerance/allergy to particular foods)

- Lying about amount or type of food consumed or evading questions about eating and weight

- Behaviors focused on food (planning, buying, preparing, and cooking meals for others but not consuming meals themselves or interest in cookbooks, recipes, and nutrition)

- Behaviors focused on body shape and weight (interest in weight-loss websites, books and magazines or images of thin people)

- Development of repetitive or obsessive behaviors relating to body shape and weight, such as pinching waist or wrists, repeated weighing, or excessive time spent looking in mirrors

- Social withdrawal or avoidance of previously enjoyed activities.

PHYSICAL WARNING SIGNS

- Weight loss or weight fluctuations

- Sensitivity to cold or feeling cold most of the time, even in warm temperatures

- Changes in menstruation

- Swelling around cheeks or jaw, calluses on knuckles, or dental discoloration from vomiting

- Fainting.

PSYCHOLOGICAL WARNING SIGNS

- Preoccupation with food, body shape, and weight

- Extreme body dissatisfaction

- Distorted body image, such as complaining of being/feeling/looking fat when actually having a healthy weight or being underweight

- Sensitivity to comments or criticism about exercise, food, body shape, or weight.

Some warning signs may be difficult to detect. This is because a person with an eating disorder

- May feel shame, guilt, and distress about eating or exercising behaviors; therefore, these will often occur in secret

- May use deceit to hide eating and exercising behaviors

- Will usually deny having a problem

- Can find it difficult to ask for help from family and friends.

Although there are many warning signs, five key signs identify a person who may have an eating disorder (see the box below). These questions give some ideas for detecting an eating disorder.[101]

The SCOFF Questionnaire[101]

QUESTIONS FOR DETECTING EATING DISORDERS

>> "Do you make yourself sick (induce vomiting) because you feel uncomfortably full?"

>> "Do you worry that you have lost control over how much you eat?"

>> "Have you recently lost more than 12 pounds in a 3-month period?"

>> "Do you think you are too fat, even though others say you are too thin?"

>> "Would you say that food dominates your life?"

For each "yes" answer, there is one point. A score of two or more indicates a likely eating disorder.

RISKS ASSOCIATED WITH EATING DISORDERS

A person with an eating disorder can experience a wide range of physical and psychological health problems. Although rapid weight loss or being very underweight is known to bring about these problems, a person does not need to be underweight for these to occur.

Severe weight loss can cause hair and nails to grow brittle and skin to dry out, become yellow, and develop a covering of soft hair. It can also slow growth and delay puberty. There can be muscle and cartilage deterioration, loss of bone density that may lead to osteoporosis and fractures, irregular or slow heartbeat, anemia, swollen joints, lightheadedness, and fainting.

Physical signs and symptoms of purging include tooth decay (due to the acid in vomit), chronically inflamed and sore throat, severe dehydration, stomach and intestinal ulcers, and inflammation of the esophagus.

Eating disorders frequently occur together with depression, anxiety disorders, and substance use disorders. When adolescents with eating disorders are followed into adulthood, most individuals recover from the eating disorder but continue to have a high level of depression and anxiety.[102]

Serious health consequences include severe malnutrition, brain dysfunction, and heart or kidney failure. The most common complications that lead to death are cardiac arrest and electrolyte and fluid imbalances. Suicide also can result.[103] Bulimia is less frequently a cause of death than anorexia; however, heart failure can occur in either disorder.

Types of Eating Disorders

Health professionals recognize three different types of eating disorders:

- Anorexia nervosa

- Bulimia nervosa

- Eating disorders not otherwise specified (EDNOS).

Anorexia Nervosa

If the person is underweight and using extreme weight-loss strategies, he or she may have anorexia nervosa. Extreme weight-loss strategies are used in an attempt to control body weight and can include dieting, fasting, overexercising, using slimming pills, diuretics, laxatives, and vomiting.

The main characteristics of anorexia nervosa are

- Overevaluation of body shape and weight, so that self-worth is largely judged in these terms

- Maintaining a very low body weight (at least 15 percent below what is considered normal for others of same height and age)

- Loss of at least three consecutive menstrual periods in females who have reached puberty

- Intense fear of gaining weight or becoming fat, even though underweight.

The overwhelming majority of people with anorexia nervosa are female. Anorexia is not common. A national survey showed that 0.6% of people had experienced anorexia nervosa some time in their life.[99] It often starts in adolescence with dieting that becomes out of control. For some people, the disorder is brief, but in others it becomes a long-term problem, and there is risk of death. People who get help early in the course of anorexia tend to have a better outcome.

Bulimia Nervosa

A person may have bulimia nervosa if they have recurrent and frequent episodes of eating unusually large amounts of food and feel a lack of control over the eating, followed by a type of behavior that compensates for the binge, such as purging, fasting, and/or excessive exercising.[103] Although by definition a person with anorexia is underweight, a person with bulimia can be slightly underweight, normal weight, or overweight.

The main characteristics of bulimia nervosa are

- Overevaluation of self by body shape or weight

- Repeated episodes of uncontrolled overeating (binge eating) for at least twice a week for 3 months or more, coupled with extreme weight control behavior (e.g., extreme dieting, frequent use of vomiting or laxatives to control weight, diuretic and enema abuse, or excessive exercise)

- Symptoms that do not meet the characteristics of anorexia.

Bulimia also mainly affects females. Bulimia often starts in adolescence or early adulthood. It is more common than anorexia. A national survey of adults found that 0.3 percent had bulimia nervosa in the previous year and 1 percent had it some time in their life.[99] It usually starts the same way as anorexia, but episodes of binge eating prevent the severe weight loss seen in anorexia. There is often a delay of many years before people with bulimia seek professional help. Approximately 16 percent of people with bulimia nervosa received treatment for mental health problems.[99]

Eating Disorders Not Otherwise Specified (EDNOS)

This category is used for people who meet some but not all the symptoms of anorexia or bulimia nervosa. People who do not fit the description of anorexia or bulimia but their attitude toward food, weight, body size, or shape is seriously interfering with their life may have another eating disorder. One example is binge-eating disorder.

BINGE-EATING DISORDER

This disorder occurs when a person has recurrent episodes of eating an unusually large amount of food in a short period of time beyond the point of feeling comfortably full. These binges occur at least twice per week over 6 months or more. The person has a sense of loss of control over his or her eating but does not use extreme weight-loss strategies to compensate. No purging is involved. Their body weight may vary from normal to overweight to obese. They often feel disgusted, distressed, ashamed, or guilty over their actions. A national survey of adults found that 1.2 percent had binge-eating disorder in the previous year and 2.8 percent had had it some time in their life.[99] Approximately 28 percent of people with binge-eating disorder received treatment for mental health problems.[99]

What Causes Eating Disorders?

As with other mental disorders, there is no single cause. A range of biological, psychological, and social factors may be contributing factors. The following factors increase a person's risk of developing an eating disorder:[104]

LIFE EXPERIENCES

- Conflict in the home, parents who have little contact with or high expectations of their children

- Sexual abuse

- Family history of dieting

- Critical comments from others about eating, weight or body shape

- Pressure to be slim because of occupation (model, jockey) or recreation (ballet, gymnastics).

PERSONAL CHARACTERISTICS

- Low self-esteem

- Perfectionism

- Anxiety

- Obesity (increases risk for bulimia)

- Early start of period in girls (increases risk for bulimia).

MENTAL DISORDERS IN FAMILY MEMBERS

- Family members with an eating disorder

- Family members with other mental disorders, such as depression, anxiety, or substance use disorders.

Importance of Early Intervention for Eating Disorders

For most people, the earlier help is sought for disordered eating and exercising behaviors, the easier it will be to overcome the problem. A delay in seeking treatment can lead to serious long-term consequences for physical and mental health. Early detection and treatment help prevent eating disorder behaviors from becoming more entrenched and increase the chance of full recovery. Anorexia and bulimia often start in adolescence. Research has shown that the sooner treatment is started, the more likely the person is to recover.[105] If a young person gets to adulthood without treatment, recovery becomes more difficult. With anorexia, there is also a high risk of death.

Mental Health First Aid Action Plan for Eating Disorders

MENTAL HEALTH FIRST AID ACTION PLAN	
ACTION A	Assess for risk of suicide or harm
ACTION L	Listen nonjudgmentally
ACTION G	Give reassurance and information
ACTION E	Encourage appropriate professional help
ACTION E®	Encourage self-help and other support strategies

ACTION A: Assess for risk of suicide or harm

Before you approach the person, learn as much as you can about eating disorders. Do this by reading books, articles, and brochures or gathering information from a reliable source, such as an eating disorder support organization or a health professional specialist. Make a plan before approaching the person; pick a place that is private, quiet, and comfortable. Avoid approaching the person in situations that may lead them to become sensitive or defensive, such as when either of you is feeling angry, emotional, tired, or frustrated or is drinking, having a meal, or in a place surrounded by food. It is better to approach the person alone, because having the whole family or a number of people confront the person at the same time could be overwhelming.

WHAT IF I DON'T FEEL COMFORTABLE TALKING TO THE PERSON?

It is common to feel nervous when approaching a person about eating and exercising behaviors. Do not avoid talking to the person because you fear it might make them angry or upset or make their problem worse. When you speak to the person, they might feel relief at having someone acknowledge their problems, or they may find it helpful to know that someone cares and has noticed that they are not coping.

WHAT SHOULD I SAY?

The way you discuss the problem will depend on the age of the person and the degree to which the problem has developed. Initially, focus on conveying empathy and not on changing the person or their perspective. Discuss your concerns in an open and honest way. Try to use "I" statements that are not accusing, such as "I am worried about you," rather than "you" statements, such as "You are making me worried." Try not to focus solely on weight or food. Rather, focus on the eating behaviors that concern you. Allow the person to discuss other concerns that are not about food, weight, or exercise. Make sure you give the person plenty of time to discuss their feelings, and reassure them it's safe to be open and honest about how they feel.

HOW WILL THE PERSON REACT?

The person may react in a variety of ways. For example, the person might be positive and receptive, they might admit they have a problem, or they might be denying, defensive, angry, or aggressive, even if you have been sensitive in your approach. The person may be relieved that someone has noticed or may seek to reassure or convince you there is no problem. They also may choose to take time to absorb your comments and concerns.

ASSESS FOR CRISES

The three main crises associated with eating disorders are

- The person has **serious health consequences**. (See box below.)

- The person has **suicidal thoughts**.

- The person is engaging in **nonsuicidal self-injury**.

Symptoms That Indicate a Physical Health Crisis[21]

- Disordered thinking and not making any reasonable sense (a person who is malnourished may appear to have psychotic symptoms such as disordered thinking, delusions, or hallucinations)

- Disorientation, doesn't know what day it is, where they are or who they are

- Vomiting several times a day

- Fainting spells

- Collapses or is too weak to walk

- Painful muscle spasms

- Chest pain or trouble breathing

- Blood in their bowel movements, urine, or vomit

- A body mass index of less than 16

- An irregular or very low heartbeat (less than 50 beats per minute)

- Cold or clammy skin indicating a low body temperature or a body temperature of less than 95 degrees Fahrenheit.

Note: A person has a right to refuse treatment, except under circumstances governed by local law, such as if the person's life is in danger.

If you have no concerns that the person is in crisis, you can ask them about how they are and move on to another Action.

Let the person know you are concerned and wish to help.

>> If you have concerns the person has **serious physical health consequences** from an eating disorder, you need to call emergency medical help. Tell the medical staff that you suspect the person has an eating disorder.

>> If there is concern about **suicidal thoughts**, see *First Aid for Suicidal Thoughts and Behaviors.*

  If you have serious concerns, call 911 or the National Suicide Prevention Lifeline at 1-800-273-TALK (8255).

>> If the person is engaging in **nonsuicidal self-injury**, see *First Aid for Nonsuicidal Self-Injury.*

ACTION L: Listen nonjudgmentally

Listen to the person's concerns, as there may be issues in his or her life that need to be identified. Depression and anxiety may also be present.

You may find it tough to listen, especially if you do not agree with what they are saying about themselves and food. It is important that you try to stay calm.

See Action L in Chapter 3 for more tips on nonjudgmental listening.

ACTION G: Give reassurance and information

Aim to provide support so that the person feels safe and secure enough to seek treatment or to talk to someone else he or she trusts (e.g., family member, friend, teacher, or coworker).

Try to see the person's behavior as related to an illness rather than to willfulness or self-indulgence.

OFFER CONSISTENT EMOTIONAL SUPPORT AND UNDERSTANDING

When talking with the person, be nonjudgmental, respectful, and kind.

Reassure the person they are deserving of your love and concern. Let them know you want them to be healthy and happy. Explain that even if there are limits to what you can do for them, you are still going to help, and you will be there to listen if they want to talk. Reassure them you are not going to take control of their life. Try not to solve their problems for them. There will be times when you don't know what to say. In this instance, just be there for the person by letting them know you care and are committed to supporting them. Avoid making promises that you cannot keep.

GIVE THE PERSON HOPE FOR RECOVERY

Reassure them that people with eating disorders can get better and that just because previous attempts to get well may have failed, it doesn't mean that they cannot get better this time. Encourage the person to be proud of any positive steps, such as acknowledging their disordered eating or exercising habits or agreeing to seek professional help.

OFFER INFORMATION

Offer to get some information about eating disorders and available help, but be careful not to overwhelm them with too much information. Remember you don't have to know all the answers, and avoid speculating about the cause.

If you become aware the person is visiting pro-ana or pro-mia websites (websites that promote eating disordered behavior), discourage further visits, as the websites can encourage destructive behavior. Be aware, however, that it is important not to mention these sites if the person is not already aware of them.

SUPPORTING THE PERSON WHO REACTS NEGATIVELY

Understand that the person may react negatively. If this happens, it is important not to take the negative reaction personally. Some reasons why the person may react negatively include the following:

- They aren't ready to make a change.

- They don't know how to change without losing their coping strategies.

- They have difficulty trusting others.

- They think you are being pushy, nosy, coercive, or bullying.

- They do not see their eating habits as a problem.

Do not express disappointment or shock if the person responds with denial, anger, aggression, tears, or defensiveness. Resist the temptation to respond angrily, as this may escalate the situation. Be willing to repeat your concerns, and remind the person that even if they don't agree, your support is still offered, and they can talk with you again in the future.

WHAT ISN'T SUPPORTIVE?

>> **Expressing negative emotion.** Arguing, being confrontational, responding angrily, or speaking harshly

>> **Saying negative things.** Criticizing, blaming, expressing disappointment or shock; trying to make the person feel ashamed or guilty; saying that what the person is doing is "disgusting" or "stupid" or "self-destructive"; making generalizations such as "you're always moody" or "you *never* do anything but exercise"

>> **Focusing on body shape or food.** Commenting positively or negatively on the person's body size or shape (e.g., "you're too thin" or "good, you've gained weight") which reinforces the idea that physical appearance is critically important to happiness or success; arguing over food or letting issues of food dominate your relationship; giving advice about weight loss, exercise, or appearance

>> **Giving simple solutions.** Saying things like "all you have to do is eat."

ACTION E: Encourage appropriate professional help

Eating disorders are complex mental disorders, and people experiencing them benefit from professional help.

DISCUSS OPTIONS FOR SEEKING PROFESSIONAL HELP

Explain that you think their behavior may indicate there is a problem that needs professional attention. Offer to assist them in getting the help they need.

If, however, the person is very underweight, he or she may not be able to take responsibility for getting professional help, as an eating disorder can affect the person's ability to think clearly.

Sometimes it is difficult for a primary care physician to assess or assist someone who is developing or experiencing an eating disorder. Not all doctors are formally trained in detecting and treating eating disorders. It is best to encourage the person to seek help from a professional with specific training in eating disorders.

PROFESSIONALS WHO CAN HELP

>> **Primary care physicians.** Doctors can diagnose an eating disorder, provide a physical checkup, give information on the physical health consequences of the disorder, refer the person to specialist mental health professionals, and link to community support.

>> **Psychiatrists and other mental health professionals.** These specialists can help the person address psychological and behavioral components of the illness.

>> **Nutritional counselors.** Nutritional experts can provide education about nutritional needs, meal planning, and monitoring eating choices.

TREATMENTS AVAILABLE FOR EATING DISORDERS

Successful treatment involves medical and psychological components. Treatment is often long-term and intensive, depending on the severity of the eating disorder. The following treatments have shown evidence of effectiveness for eating disorders:

>> **Anorexia.** There has been little research on what treatments work best. The first goal for treatment is to ensure the person's physical health, which involves restoring the person to a healthy weight. Sometimes it is necessary to admit the person to a hospital, depending upon how excessive the weight loss. There are no medications proven to work with anorexia. However, one treatment that is known to work for adolescents with anorexia is family therapy in which the parents are encouraged to take control of feeding their child and to prevent severe dieting, purging, and overexercise.

>> **Bulimia.** Cognitive behavioral therapy is generally the most effective treatment. It aims to change eating habits and weight control behaviors, as well as the person's preoccupation with body shape and weight.

Another treatment that works is interpersonal psychotherapy. In this treatment, the emphasis is on helping the person to identify and change interpersonal problems that contribute to an eating disorder.

Antidepressants can also help with bulimia but are not as effective as cognitive behavioral therapy (CBT).

>> **Binge eating disorder.** CBT is also effective for binge-eating disorder. Interpersonal psychotherapy and antidepressants can also help, but the evidence for their effectiveness is not as strong as for CBT.

WHAT IF THE PERSON DOESN'T WANT HELP?

People with an eating disorder may refuse professional help. In a national survey of people with eating disorders, less than a third had received treatment in the previous 12 months.[99] Understand that the person may resist help for a number of reasons (see the following box).

Reasons the Person May Resist Help

The person may

- Feel ashamed of his or her behavior

- Fear gaining weight or losing control over his or her weight

- Be afraid of acknowledging that he or she is unwell

- Not think that he or she is ill

- Believe there are benefits to their disordered eating or exercising behaviors; controlling their weight may make them feel better about themselves or provide a sense of accomplishment.

Try not to expect the person to immediately follow your advice. Remember, you cannot force the person to change or to seek help. If the person is resistant, continue to suggest professional help, while being sensitive toward the person's fears about the process. In the meantime, seek advice from an organization that specializes in eating disorders.

Recognize that eating disorders are long-term problems that are not easily overcome.

Although you may feel frustrated by the person's behavior, it is important you do not threaten to end your relationship with the person. Rather than giving up on the person, continue to be supportive, positive, and encouraging while you are waiting for him or her to accept the need to change. Be encouraging of the person's strengths and interests unrelated to food or physical appearance. Acknowledge the person's positive attributes, successes, and accomplishments, and try to view the person as an individual rather than just someone who has an eating disorder.

ACTION E: Encourage self-help and other support strategies

OTHER PEOPLE WHO CAN HELP
You can suggest that the person surround himself or herself with supportive people. There are organizations that provide information and support for people with eating disorders (see Helpful Resources).

SELF-HELP STRATEGIES[106]
Self-help books based on CBT can work for bulimia and binge-eating disorder. It is best to work through these books under the guidance of a therapist, but there is also benefit in using these books as self-help.

Helpful Resources

FOR EATING DISORDERS

WEB SITES

Mental Health America

www.mentalhealthamerica.net

Visit Mental Health America's site for information on mental health, getting help, and taking action.

National Association of Anorexia Nervosa and Associated Disorders

www.anad.org

This site includes information about eating disorders, how to seek treatment, and support groups for people suffering from eating disorders and their families.

National Council for Behavioral Health

www.TheNationalCouncil.org

To locate mental health and addictions treatment facilities in your community, use the Find a Provider feature on the National Council's website.

National Eating Disorders Association

www.nationaleatingdisorders.org

This site has stories of recovery from eating disorders, information about seeking treatment, and additional resources for school professionals and caregivers.

National Institute of Mental Health

www.nimh.nih.gov

The National Institute of Mental Health website has links to information about eating disorders.

Something Fishy

www.somethingfishy.org

This website provides useful information and links for those with an eating disorder or friends and families. It also has online support options such as web boards and links to chat rooms.

Substance Abuse and Mental Health Services Administration

www.samhsa.gov

This website has links to information about eating disorders.

BOOKS

Fairburn, C. (1995) *Overcoming binge eating.* Guilford Press, New York, NY.
This self-help manual may help people who are struggling with binge-eating disorder and bulimia nervosa to gain control over their eating.

McCabe, R. E., McFarlane, T. L., and Olmstead, M. P. (2004) *Overcoming bulimia: your comprehensive, step-by-step guide to recovery.* New Harbinger Publications, Oakland, CA.
This self-help workbook uses the principles of cognitive behavior therapy to help people with bulimia help themselves.

Schaefer, J., and Rutledge, T. (2003) *Life without Ed: how one woman declared independence from her eating disorder and how you can too.* McGraw-Hill, Columbus, OH.
Written by a woman who recovered from fluctuating episodes of anorexia nervosa and bulimia nervosa, with contributions by her therapist, this book details the difficult road to discovery. "Ed" is the name given to the eating disorder.

Gürze Books

www.gurze.com

This website offers all types of books on eating disorders. Listed are self-help books, many based on cognitive behavioral therapy; information for people with eating disorders, their families, and therapists; and autobiographical books documenting recovery from an eating disorder.

SUPPORT GROUPS

American Self-Help Group Clearinghouse

www.mentalhelp.net/selfhelp/

This searchable database lists 1,100 self-help and caregiver support groups, including many for eating disorders. Also listed are local self-help clearinghouses worldwide, research studies, information on starting face-to-face and online groups, and a registry for persons interested in starting national or international self-help groups.

Eating Disorders Anonymous

www.eatingdisordersanonymous.org

Following the 12-step approach used by Alcoholics Anonymous, Eating Disorders Anonymous can help people struggling with eating disorders. The website lists meetings nationwide.

Overeaters Anonymous

www.oa.org

Following the 12-step approach used by Alcoholics Anonymous, Overeaters Anonymous can help people struggling with compulsive eating and binge eating. The website lists Overeaters Anonymous meetings nationwide.

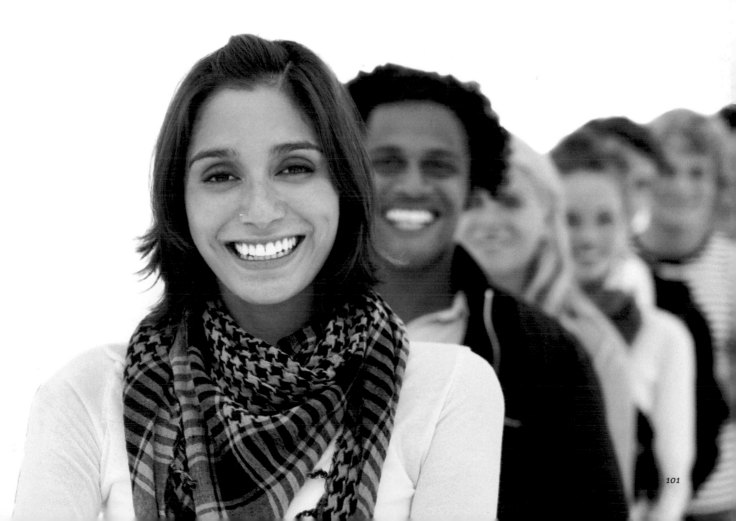

SECTION THREE: FIRST AID FOR MENTAL HEALTH CRISES

This section contains recommendations on how to give first aid in a number of mental health crisis situations. Some of these crises can occur in people with various mental disorders or those in emotional distress. Others may precipitate the onset of a mental disorder or may be related to substance use. The role of the first aider is to assist the person until appropriate professional help is received or the crisis resolves.

The first aid advice in this section is based on international guidelines that have been developed using the expert consensus of panels of mental health consumers, caregivers, and clinicians. These experts came from a range of developed English-speaking countries: Australia, Canada, Ireland, New Zealand, the United Kingdom, and the United States.

Each individual is unique, and it is important to tailor your support to that person's needs. These recommendations therefore may not be appropriate for every person in crisis.

Recommendations are provided for the following situations:

1. Suicidal thoughts and behaviors

2. Nonsuicidal self-injury

3. Panic attacks

4. Traumatic events affecting adults

5. Traumatic events affecting children

6. Acute psychosis

7. Medical emergency from alcohol abuse

8. Aggressive behavior

CHAPTER 8

First Aid for Mental Health Crises

① First Aid for Suicidal Thoughts and Behaviors[38, 107]

An important note

Self-injury can indicate a number of different things. Someone who is hurting himself or herself may be at risk of suicide. Others engage in a pattern of self-injury over weeks, months, or years and are not necessarily suicidal. This advice can be of use to you only if the person is suicidal. If the person you are assisting is injuring himself or herself but is not suicidal, please refer to *First Aid for Nonsuicidal Self-Injury*.

How Can I Tell if Someone Is Feeling Suicidal?[45]

It is important that you know the warning signs of suicide.

Signs a person may be suicidal:

- Threatening to hurt or kill himself or herself

- Looking for ways to kill himself or herself: seeking access to pills, weapons, or other means

- Talking or writing about death, dying, or suicide

- Hopelessness

- Rage, anger, seeking revenge

- Acting recklessly or engaging in risky activities, seemingly without thinking

- Feeling trapped, like there's no way out

- Increasing alcohol or drug use

- Withdrawing from friends, family, or society

- Anxiety, agitation, unable to sleep or sleeping all the time

- Dramatic changes in mood

- No reason for living, no sense of purpose in life.

People may show one or many of these signs, and some may show signs not on this list.

If you suspect someone may be at risk for suicide, it is important to ask directly about suicidal thoughts. Do not avoid using the word "suicide." It is important to ask the question without dread and without expressing a negative judgment. The question must be direct and to the point. For example, you could ask

- *Are you having thoughts of suicide?*

- *Are you thinking about killing yourself?*

If you appear confident in the face of a suicide crisis, this can be reassuring for the suicidal person.

Although some people think talking about suicide can plant the idea in the person's mind, this is not true. Another myth is that someone who talks about suicide isn't really serious. Remember that talking about suicide may be a way to indicate just how badly the person is feeling.

How should I talk with someone who is suicidal?

It is important to do the following:

- Tell the person that you care and that you want to help.

- Express empathy.

- Clearly state that thoughts of suicide are often associated with a treatable mental disorder, as this may instill a sense of hope.

- Tell the person that thoughts of suicide are common and do not have to be acted on.

Suicidal thoughts are often a plea for help and a desperate attempt to escape from problems and distressing feelings. Encourage the suicidal person to do most of the talking, if they are able. They need the opportunity to talk about their feelings and reasons for wanting to die, and they may feel great relief at being able to do this.

It may be helpful to talk about specific problems the person is experiencing. Discuss ways to deal with issues that seem impossible, but do not attempt to solve the problems yourself.

How can I tell if the situation is serious?

First, you need to determine whether the person has definite intentions to take their life or if their thoughts are more vague, such as "What's the point of going on?" To do this, you need to ask the person if they have a plan for suicide. The three questions you need to ask are

1. Have you decided how you would kill yourself?

2. Have you decided when you would do it?

3. Have you taken any steps to secure the things you would need to carry out your plan?

A higher level of planning indicates a more serious risk. However, you must remember that the absence of a plan is not enough to ensure the person's safety. All thoughts of suicide must be taken seriously.

Next, you need to know about the following extra risk factors:

- Has the person been using alcohol or other drugs? Such use can make a person more susceptible to acting on impulse.

- Has the person made a suicide attempt in the past? A previous attempt makes a person more likely to try again or complete suicide. Once you have established the risk of suicide is present, you need to take action to keep the person safe.

How can I keep the person safe?

A person who is actively suicidal should not be left alone. If you can't stay, you need to arrange for someone else to do so. In addition, give the person a safety contact that is available at all times (such as a telephone help line, a friend or family member who has agreed to help, or a mental health professional).

It is important to help the person think about people or things that have helped in the past. These might include a doctor, psychologist, or other mental health worker; family member or friend; or a community group such as a club or church.

Do not use guilt and threats to prevent suicide (e.g., "You will go to hell").

What about professional help?

›› During the crisis. Mental health professionals advocate always asking for professional help when a person is suicidal, especially if the person is psychotic. If the person who is suicidal has a weapon or is behaving aggressively toward you, you must seek assistance from law enforcement to protect yourself.

However, the person may be very reluctant to involve a professional, and if the person is close to you, you may be concerned about alienating them. In fact, some people who have experienced suicidal thoughts or who have made plans for suicide feel that professional help is not always necessary.

›› After the crisis has passed. Ensure the person gets needed psychological and medical help. Other parts of this manual may be useful for you in achieving this.

What if the person makes me promise not to tell anyone else?

Never agree to keep someone's plan for suicide a secret. However, respect the person's right to privacy, and involve him or her in decisions regarding who else knows about his or her suicidal intentions.

The person I am trying to help has injured himself or herself but insists he or she is not suicidal. What should I do?

Some people injure themselves for reasons other than suicide. This may be to relieve unbearable anguish, to stop feeling numb, or other reasons. This can be distressing to see. *First Aid for Nonsuicidal Self-Injury* can help you to understand and assist if this is occurring.

A final note

Do your best for the person, but remember that despite our best efforts, some people will still die by suicide.

② First Aid for Nonsuicidal Self-Injury[108, 109]

An important note

This first aid advice applies only if the person is injuring himself or herself for reasons other than suicide. If the person you are assisting is injuring himself or herself and is suicidal, please refer to *First Aid for Suicidal Thoughts and Behaviors*.

Facts on Nonsuicidal Self-Injury[46]

Many terms are used to describe self-injury, such as *self-harm, self-mutilation, cutting,* and *parasuicide.* There is a great deal of debate about what self-injury is and how it is different from suicidal behavior. Here the term *nonsuicidal self-injury* is used to refer to situations where the self-injury has no suicidal intent. It is not easy to tell the difference between nonsuicidal self-injury and a suicide attempt. The only way to know is to ask the person directly if they are suicidal.

There are many different types of nonsuicidal self-injury, including

- Cutting, scratching, or pinching skin enough to cause bleeding or a mark that remains on the skin

- Banging or punching objects to the point of bruising or bleeding

- Ripping and tearing skin

- Carving words or patterns into skin

- Interfering with the healing of wounds

- Burning skin with cigarettes, matches, or hot water

- Pulling out large amounts of hair

- Deliberately overdosing on medications when this is *not* meant as a suicide attempt.

Nonsuicidal self-injury is relatively common in young people. A survey of U.S. college students found that 17 percent had engaged in nonsuicidal self-injury at some time in their lives.[46] Another survey of high school students found that 20 percent of girls and 9 percent of boys had engaged in nonsuicidal self-injury. These young people reported more emotional distress, more anger problems, lower self-esteem, more risky health behaviors, and more antisocial behaviors.[47]

People who engage in nonsuicidal self-injury do so for many reasons, including to[48]

- Escape from unbearable anguish

- Change the behavior of others

- Escape from a situation

- Show desperation to others

- "Get back at" other people or make them feel guilty

- Gain relief of tension

- Seek attention or help.

Recent research has found that adolescents have engaged in nonsuicidal self-injury if they have close friends or peers who engage in similar behaviors.[49]

How should I talk with someone who is deliberately injuring?

If you suspect that someone you care about is deliberately self-injuring, you need to discuss it. If you have noticed suspicious injuries on the person's body, do not ignore it. Instead, let the person know that you have noticed. Avoid expressing a strong negative reaction to the self-injury, and discuss it calmly. It is important that you have reflected on your own state of mind and are prepared to nonjudgmentally deal with the answer.

Understand that self-injury is a coping mechanism, and therefore stopping self-injury should not be the focus of the conversation. Instead, look at ways to relieve the distress. Do not trivialize the feelings or situations that have led to the self-injury. Do not punish the person, especially by threatening to withdraw care.

What should I do if I witness someone deliberately injuring?

If you have interrupted someone in the act of deliberate self-injury, intervene in a supportive and nonjudgmental way. Remain calm and avoid expressions of shock or anger. Express your concern for the person's well-being. Ask whether you can do anything to alleviate the distress. Ask if medical attention is needed.

What about professional help?

›› Medical emergency. If the person has taken an overdose of medication or consumed poison, call an ambulance. Deliberate overdose is more frequently intended as a suicide attempt but is sometimes a form of self-injury. Regardless of the person's intentions, emergency medical help must be sought.

If the injury is life-threatening, seek emergency medical help. Emergency services should be called if the person is confused, disoriented, unconscious, or has bleeding that is rapid or pulsing.

›› Obtaining mental health care. Encourage the person to seek professional help. Self-injury is not an illness but a symptom of mental illness or serious psychological distress that needs treatment. Ensure the person knows where to obtain professional mental health care, but do not force the issue.

Further information about encouraging a person to seek professional treatment can be found in the other guidelines in this series.

How can I keep the person safe?

Encourage the person to speak to someone he or she trusts the next time he or she feels the urge to self-injure. Also, ensure first aid supplies are accessible to the person.

③ First Aid for Panic Attacks[110]

Facts on Panic Attacks[21]

More than one in five people experience at least one panic attack in their lifetime, but few go on to develop panic disorder or agoraphobia (anxiety disorders related to panic attacks).[56]

A panic attack is a distinct episode of high anxiety with fear or discomfort. The attack develops abruptly and has its peak within 10 minutes. During the attack, several of the following symptoms are present:

■ Palpitations, pounding heart, rapid heart rate

■ Sweating

■ Trembling and shaking

■ Shortness of breath, sensations of choking or smothering

■ Chest pain or discomfort

■ Abdominal distress or nausea

■ Dizziness, lightheadedness, feeling faint or unsteady

■ Feelings of unreality or being detached from oneself

■ Fears of losing control or going crazy

■ Fear of dying

■ Numbness or tingling

■ Chills or hot flashes.

What should I do if I think someone is having a panic attack?

If someone is experiencing these symptoms and you suspect a panic attack, ask if the person knows what is happening or has previously had a panic attack. If they have had a previous panic attack and believe that they are having one now, ask if they need help and give it to them. If you are helping someone you do not know, introduce yourself.

What if I am uncertain whether the person is really having a panic attack and not something more serious like a heart attack?

Symptoms of a panic attack sometimes resemble a heart attack or other medical problem. It is not possible to be totally sure; only a medical professional can tell if it is something more serious. If the person has not had a prior panic attack and doesn't think he or she is having one now, follow physical first aid guidelines.

Ask the person, or check for a medical alert bracelet or necklace. Follow the instructions on the alert or seek medical assistance.

If the person loses consciousness, apply physical first aid principles. Check for breathing and pulse and call an ambulance.

What should I say and do if I know the person is having a panic attack?

Reassure the person that he or she is experiencing a panic attack. It is important you remain calm and do not start to panic yourself. Speak to the person in a reassuring but firm manner, and be patient. Speak clearly and slowly and use short, clear sentences.

Rather than making assumptions about what the person needs, ask him or her directly what they think might help.

Do not belittle the person's experience. Acknowledge that the terror feels very real, but reassure them that a panic attack, while frightening, is not life-threatening or dangerous. Reassure them that they are safe and that the symptoms will pass.

What should I say and do when the panic attack has ended?

After the attack has subsided, ask if they know where they can get information about panic attacks. If they don't know, offer suggestions.

Tell the person that if the panic attack recurs and is causing them distress, he or she should speak to an appropriate health professional. Become knowledgeable about the range of professional help available for panic attacks in your community. Reassure the person that there are effective treatments available for panic attacks and panic disorder.

What should I do if the person is breathing rapidly?

Breathing rapidly is common when an individual is experiencing a panic attack. Do not force the person to focus on slowing their breathing. Instead, remain calm and model a normal breathing rate.

A common myth is to recommend having the person breathe into a paper bag in order to slow their breathing. Breathing into a bag causes the person to inhale their own carbon dioxide, which may cause the person to become unconscious.[117]

④ First Aid for Adults Affected by Traumatic Events[111]

Facts on Traumatic Events

A traumatic event is any incident experienced by the person that is perceived to be traumatic. Common examples of traumas that affect individuals include accidents (such as traffic or physical accidents), assault (including physical or sexual assault, mugging or robbery, or family violence), and witnessing something terrible happen. Mass traumatic events include terrorist attacks, mass shootings, and severe weather events (such as hurricane, tsunami, or forest fire).

Mental health first aid might not always be possible immediately after the traumatic event. Sometimes, trauma is not a single incident, and mental health first aid should be administered when the first aider becomes aware of the problem:

■ Recurring trauma includes sexual, physical, or emotional abuse; torture; and bullying in the schoolyard or workplace.

■ Memories of a traumatic event suddenly or unexpectedly return weeks, months, or even years afterwards, causing distress.

It is important to know that people can differ in how they react to traumatic events:

■ One person may perceive an event as deeply traumatic, while another does not.

■ Particular types of traumas affect some individuals more than others.

■ A history of trauma may make some people more susceptible to later traumatic events, while others become more resilient.

What are the first priorities for helping someone after a traumatic event?

Ensure your own safety before offering help to anyone. Check for potential dangers, such as fire, weapons, debris, or other people who may become aggressive, before deciding to approach a person to offer help.

If you are helping someone whom you do not know, introduce yourself and explain your role. Find out the person's name and use it when talking. Remain calm, and do what you can to create a safe environment by taking the person to a safer location or removing any immediate danger.

If the person is injured, it is important to get treatment. If you are able, offer the person first aid and seek medical assistance. If the person seems unhurt, you need to watch for changes in his or her physical or mental state and be prepared to seek emergency medical assistance. Be aware that a person may suddenly become disoriented or may have internal injuries that reveal themselves more slowly.

Determine what the person's immediate needs are for food, water, shelter, or clothing. If there are professional helpers nearby (police, ambulance, or others) who are better able to meet those needs, don't take over their role.

If the person has been a victim of assault, you need to consider the possibility that forensic evidence may need to be collected (such as cheek swabs or evidence on clothing or skin). Work to preserve such evidence where possible. For example, they may want to change their clothes and shower, which may destroy forensic evidence. It may be helpful to put clothing in a bag for law enforcement to take as evidence and suggest to the person that they wait to shower until after a forensic exam. Although collecting evidence is important, you should not force the person to do anything they don't want to do.

Do not make promises you may not be able to keep. For example, don't say you will get the person home soon if this is not possible or likely.

What are the priorities if I am helping after a mass traumatic event?

Mass traumatic events are those that affect large numbers of people. They include severe environmental events (such as fires and floods), acts of war and terrorism, and mass shootings. In addition to the general principles outlined above, there are a number of things you need to do:

>> **Find out what emergency help is available.** If there are professional helpers at the scene, follow their directions.

>> **Be responsive to the comfort and dignity of the person you are helping.** Offer a blanket or coat to cover them, or ask bystanders or media to move away. Try not to appear rushed or impatient.

>> **Give truthful information, but admit when you don't know something, as well.** Tell the person about information sources offered to victims, such as information sessions, fact sheets, and special telephone information help lines, as they become available. Don't give the person any information he or she does not want to hear, as this can be traumatic in itself.

How do I talk to someone who has just experienced a traumatic event?

When talking to a person who has experienced a traumatic event, it is more important to be genuinely caring than to say the right things. Show the person that you understand and care, and ask how you can best help. Speak clearly and avoid clinical and technical language, and communicate with the person as an equal, rather than as a superior or expert. If the person seems unable to understand, you may need to calmly repeat yourself. Providing support doesn't have to be complicated; it can involve small things like spending time with the person, having a cup of tea or coffee, chatting about day-to-day life, or giving a hug.

Behavior such as withdrawal, irritability, and bad temper may be a response to the trauma, so try not to take such behavior personally. Be friendly, even if the person is being difficult.

The person may not be as distressed about what has happened as you might expect, and this is fine. Don't tell them how they should be feeling. Tell them that everyone deals with trauma at their own pace. Be aware that cultural differences may influence the way some people respond; for example, in some cultures, expressing vulnerability or grief around strangers is not considered appropriate.

Should we talk about what happened? How can I support someone in doing so?

It is very important you do not force the person to talk. Remember, you are not the person's therapist.

Encourage the person to talk about his or her reactions only if they feel ready. If the person does want to talk, don't interrupt to share your own feelings, experiences, or opinions. Be aware that the person may need to talk repetitively about the trauma, so you may need to be willing to listen on more than one occasion.

Avoid saying anything that might trivialize the person's feelings, such as "don't cry" or "calm down," or anything that minimizes his or her experience, such as "you should just be glad you're alive."

The person might experience survivor guilt, the feeling that it is unfair that others died or were injured when the person was not.

How can I help the person to cope over the next few weeks or months?

If you are helping someone you don't know, unless you are responsible for them in some professional capacity, it is not expected that you will have further contact. If it is someone close to you, such as a friend or family member, your support can be very helpful.

Encourage the person to tell others when he or she needs or wants something rather than relying on assumptions. Also encourage him or her to identify sources of support, including loved ones and friends, but remember that it is important to respect the person's need to be alone at times.

Encourage the person to get plenty of rest, and to do things that feel good (such as take baths, read, exercise, or watch television). Encourage them to think about coping strategies they have successfully used in the past and to spend time where they feel safe and comfortable.

Be aware the person may suddenly or unexpectedly remember details of the event and may or may not wish to discuss these details. If this happens, the general principles outlined above can help you to assist the person.

Discourage the person from using negative coping strategies such as working too hard, using alcohol and other drugs, or engaging in self-destructive behavior.

When should the person seek professional help?

Not everyone will need professional help to recover from a traumatic event. If the person wants to seek help, offer your support. Be aware of professional help that is available locally, and if the person does not like the first professional they speak to, tell them that it is okay to try a different one. If the person hasn't indicated that they want professional help, the following guidelines can help you to determine whether help is needed.

If at any time the person becomes suicidal, seek professional help. *First Aid for Suicidal Thoughts and Feelings* may be useful in helping you to do this. Also, if at any time the person abuses alcohol or other drugs to deal with the trauma, encourage professional help.

After four weeks, some return to normal functioning is expected. Encourage professional help if, for four weeks or longer after the trauma, they

- Are still very upset or fearful

- Seem unable to escape intense, ongoing feelings of distress

- Withdraw from family or friends and/or important relationships are suffering

- Feel jumpy or have trauma-related nightmares

- Can't stop thinking about the trauma

- Are unable to enjoy life at all

- Have posttrauma symptoms that are interfering with usual activities.

⑤ First Aid for Children Affected by Traumatic Events[112]

What are the first priorities for helping a child after a traumatic event?

You need to ensure your own safety before offering help. Determine whether it is safe to approach the child. Check for potential dangers like fire, weapons, or falling debris, and watch for other people who might become aggressive.

If you are helping a child you do not know, introduce yourself and explain that you are there to help. Find out the child's name and use it when talking him or her. Remain calm. Do what you can to ensure safety by taking the child to a safer location or removing any immediate dangers. Reassure the child that he or she won't be left alone. Ensure that you or another adult (such as a professional helper) are available to take care of the child. If you have to leave the child alone for a few minutes to attend to others, reassure the child that you will be back soon. Try not to behave in such a way that the child feels he or she is still in danger.

If the child is hurt, it is important to attend to his or her injuries. If you are able, give the child first aid and seek medical assistance. If the child seems uninjured, you need to watch for a change in physical or mental state, and be prepared to seek emergency medical assistance. Be aware the child may suddenly become disoriented, or an apparently uninjured child may have internal injuries that reveal themselves more slowly.

Try to determine what the child's immediate needs are for food, water, shelter, or clothing. However, if there are professional helpers nearby (police, ambulance, or others) who are better able to meet those needs, don't take over their role.

Don't make promises you may not be able to keep. For example, don't promise the child can go home soon, when this may not be the case.

What are the priorities if I am helping after a mass traumatic event?

Mass traumatic events are those that affect large numbers of people. They include severe environmental events (such as fires and floods), acts of war and terrorism, and mass shootings. In addition to the more general guidelines above, there are a number of things you need to do.

Try to keep the child together with any loved ones and caregivers who are present. If they are not present or have been separated from the child in the course of the event, ensure that the child is reconnected as soon as possible.

Ask the child what would make him or her feel better or safer. Direct the child away from traumatic sights and sounds, including media images, and people who are injured or distressed, such as anyone who is screaming, agitated, or aggressive. Ask bystanders and the media to stay away from the child.

How do I talk to a child who has experienced a traumatic event?

This advice may be used to help you support a child after a traumatic event. If you know the child, you can use these guidelines to offer ongoing support at home or in a classroom. If you don't know the child, use these guidelines at the scene of the trauma or in any future contact you may have with the child.

Remember, when talking to a child who has experienced a traumatic event, it is more important to be genuinely caring than to say the right things. Show the child you understand and care, and tell the child you will do your best to ensure safety.

Talk to the child using age-appropriate language and explanations. Allow the child to ask questions and answer as truthfully as possible. Be patient if the child asks the same question many times, and try to be consistent with answers and information. If you can't answer a question, admit to the child that you don't know the answer.

If the child knows accurate, upsetting details, don't deny these. When someone has died, it can be tempting to soften this news by telling a child that the person has "gone to sleep." Avoid this, as it may make the child fearful of sleep.

A child may stop talking altogether after a trauma. If this happens, don't try to force the child to speak. Equally, you should never coerce a child to talk about feelings or memories of the trauma before he or she is ready.

If the child wants to talk about his or her feelings, allow it, but remember that some children prefer to express their feelings through writing, drawing, or playing with toys.

Never tell the child how to feel. Don't tell the child to be brave or not to cry, and don't make judgments about their feelings. Don't get angry if the child expresses strong emotions; instead, tell them it is okay to feel upset when something bad or scary happens.

A child has told me that they are being abused. What should I do?

Remain calm and reassure the child they have done the right thing by telling you and that what happened was not their fault. Tell the child that you believe them.

You need to know the local laws on reporting suspected child abuse and follow these. Contact the appropriate authorities, and work with them to ensure the child's safety. Do not confront the perpetrator.

I am a parent/guardian, and the child I am helping lives with me. How should I behave at home?

Try to keep your behavior as predictable as possible, and tell the child that you (and other loved ones) love and support them. Encourage them to do things they enjoy, such as playing with toys or reading books. You can help the child to feel in control by letting them make some decisions, such as choosing what to eat or wear.

>> **Dealing with temper tantrums and avoidance behaviors.** Be aware the child may avoid things that remind them of the trauma, such as specific places, riding in the car, certain people, or separation from parents or guardians. Try to figure out what triggers fearfulness or regression in the child. If the child has temper tantrums or becomes fearful, crying and clingy in order to avoid reminders of the trauma, ask them what scares them. Don't get angry or call the child "babyish" if they appear to regress by bedwetting, misbehaving, or sucking their thumb.

If the child avoids reminders of the trauma but does not appear very distressed, ask what they are afraid of and assure them that they are safe.

The symptoms associated with trauma may suddenly or unexpectedly appear months or years after the event. If this occurs, professional help may need to be sought.

Should the child receive professional help?

Not all children will need professional help to recover from a traumatic event. The following guidelines can help you determine whether help is needed.

If at any time the child becomes suicidal, seek immediate professional help.

Seek professional help if, for two weeks or more after the trauma, the child

- Is unable to enjoy life at all

- Displays sudden severe or delayed reactions to trauma

- Is unable to escape intense ongoing distressing feelings

- Has post trauma symptoms that interfere with their usual activities

- Withdraws from caregivers or friends, or other important relationships are suffering.

Seek professional help if, four weeks or more after the trauma, the child

- Experiences temper tantrums or becomes fearful, crying, and clingy in order to avoid reminders of the event

- Still feels very upset or fearful

- Acts or behaves very differently compared to before the trauma

- Feels jumpy or has nightmares because of or about the trauma

- Can't stop thinking about the trauma.

Become knowledgeable about the types of professional help that are available locally for children. Clinical child psychologists, psychiatrists, pediatricians, and family doctors can all be helpful. If you are not the child's parent or guardian, do not seek professional help unless it is an emergency; instead, assist the child's parent or guardian to seek professional help.

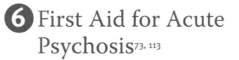

❻ First Aid for Acute Psychosis[73, 113]

Facts on Acute Psychosis

A person who is experiencing psychosis may have difficulty distinguishing what is real and what is not. Psychosis can occur as part of a number of mental disorders such as schizophrenia or bipolar disorder or when a person is intoxicated with a drug. In acute psychosis, the person has severe symptoms such as delusions, hallucinations, very disorganized thinking, and odd behaviors. They may be unable to care for themselves appropriately. The person's behavior is disruptive or disturbing to others, prompting them to seek assistance for the person's symptoms.

What should I do in a crisis situation when the person has become acutely unwell?

In a crisis situation, remain as calm as possible. Evaluate the situation by assessing the risks involved,

such as whether the person will harm self or others. It is important to assess whether the person is at risk of suicide. For advice on how to do this, refer to *First Aid for Suicidal Thoughts and Behavior*. If the person has an advance directive or relapse prevention plan, follow those instructions. Try to find out if the person has trusted friends or family, and enlist their help. Assess whether it is safe for the person to be alone, and if not, ensure that someone stays with him or her.

It is important to communicate in a clear and concise manner and use short, simple sentences. Speak quietly in a nonthreatening tone of voice at a moderate pace. If the person asks you questions, answer calmly. Comply with requests unless they are unsafe or unreasonable. This gives the person the opportunity to feel somewhat in control.

Be aware that the person might act upon a delusion or hallucination. Remember that your primary task is to de-escalate the situation, and therefore don't do anything to further agitate the person. Try to maintain safety and protect the person, yourself, and others from harm. Make sure you have access to an exit if you feel in danger.

You may not be able to de-escalate the situation, and if this is the case, be prepared to call for assistance. If the person is at risk of harming self or others, make sure he or she is evaluated by a medical or mental health professional immediately. When the crisis staff arrives, you should convey specific, concise observations about the severity of the person's behavior and symptoms. You should explain to the person that the unfamiliar people are there to help and describe how they are going to help. If your concerns about the person are dismissed by the services you contact, you should persevere in trying to seek support.

What if the person becomes aggressive?

People with psychosis are not usually aggressive and are more likely to harm themselves than others. However, hallucinations and delusions can occasionally cause people with psychosis to become aggressive. If this occurs, follow the advice in *First Aid for Aggressive Behavior*.

❼ First Aid for a Medical Emergency from Alcohol Abuse[114]

Facts on Alcohol Intoxication, Poisoning, and Withdrawal

>> **Alcohol intoxication** refers to significantly elevated levels of alcohol in a person's bloodstream, which substantially impair the person's thinking and behavior.

>> **Alcohol poisoning** means the person has a toxic level of alcohol in the bloodstream. This can lead to death. The amount of alcohol that causes alcohol poisoning is different for every person.

>> **Alcohol withdrawal** refers to the aversive symptoms a person experiences when they stop drinking or drink substantially less than usual. Alcohol withdrawal, without the aid of medication, may lead to seizures.

The Recovery Position[118]

Any unconscious person needs *immediate medical attention* and their *airway kept open*.

If left lying on their back, they could suffocate on their vomit, or their tongue could block their airways. Putting the person in the recovery position will help to keep the airway open.

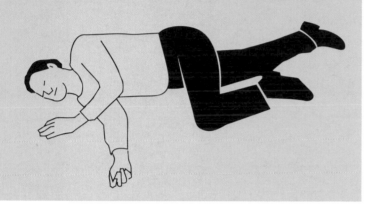

If the person is intoxicated,

>> **Stay calm.**

>> **Communicate appropriately.** Talk in a respectful manner and use simple, clear language. Do not laugh at, make fun of, or provoke the person.

>> **Monitor for danger.** While intoxicated, the person may engage in a wide range of risky activities, such as having unprotected sex, vandalizing property, or driving. Assess the situation for potential danger, and ensure that everyone is safe. Monitor the person and the environment to prevent tripping or falling. Ask if they have taken any medications or other drugs, in case their condition deteriorates into a medical emergency.

>> **Ensure the person's safety.** Do not leave the person alone. Be aware the person may be more intoxicated than they realize. Keep them away from machines and dangerous objects. If the

person attempts to drive (or ride a bike), try to discourage them by telling them about the risks to self and others. Only prevent the person from driving if it is safe for you to do so. If it is unsafe, call law enforcement. Arrange for the person to go to a hospital if the person is a risk; otherwise, organize a safe mode of transport home.

Can I help the person sober up?

Only time will reverse the effects of intoxication. The body metabolizes approximately one standard drink of alcohol an hour. Drinking black coffee, sleeping, walking, and cold showers will not speed this process.

ALCOHOL INTOXICATION, POISONING, AND WITHDRAWAL MAY LEAD TO A MEDICAL EMERGENCY

See box on the next page on *when to call an ambulance* for more information on symptoms to look for. If the person appears at risk of a medical emergency, ensure that

■ An ambulance is called or medical help sought— do not be afraid to seek medical help, even if there may be legal implications for the person

■ The person is not left alone

■ The person's airway, breathing, and circulation are monitored

■ If the person is hard to wake, place him or her in the recovery position—see box on *The Recovery Position* for more information

■ Broken glass and other sharp objects are kicked out of the way before rolling the person into the recovery position

■ No food is given to the person, as he or she may choke on it if they are not fully conscious

- The person is kept warm to prevent hypothermia—although the person may feel warm, body temperature may be decreasing.

ADDITIONAL FIRST AID PRINCIPLES:

- Be aware that alcohol consumption can mask pain from injuries.

- If the person is vomiting and conscious, keep the person sitting. Alternatively, put them in the recovery position. If necessary, clear their airway after they have vomited.

- If the person stops breathing, he or she will need expired air resuscitation (EAR).

- If the person has no pulse, he or she will need cardiopulmonary resuscitation (CPR).

- It can be beneficial for a friend or family member to accompany the person to the hospital, as they may be able to provide relevant information.

When to Call an Ambulance

Do not be afraid to seek medical help for the person, even if there may be legal implications. It may be beneficial for a friend or family member to accompany the person to the hospital, as they may be able to provide relevant information.

Call an ambulance or seek medical help if the person

- Cannot be awakened or is unconscious

- Has irregular, shallow, or slow breathing

- Has irregular, weak, or slow pulse rate

- Has cold, clammy, pale, or bluish skin

- Is continually vomiting

- Shows signs of a possible head injury (e.g., vomiting, talking incoherently)

- Has seizures

- Has delirium tremens—a state of confusion and visual hallucinations

- Has convulsions

- Has blackouts—when the person forgets what happened during the drinking episode

- May have consumed a spiked drink.

What do I do if the intoxicated person becomes aggressive?

If this occurs, follow the advice in *First Aid for Aggressive Behavior*.

⑧ First Aid for Aggressive Behavior[73, 113, 114]

If the person becomes aggressive, ensure your own safety at all times. Remain as calm as possible, and try to de-escalate the situation.

How to De-escalate the Situation

- Speak to the person slowly and confidently with a gentle, caring tone of voice.

- Do not respond in a hostile, disciplinary, or challenging manner.

- Do not argue.

- Do not threaten, as this may increase fear or prompt aggressive behavior.

- Avoid raising your voice or talking too fast.

- Be aware the person may overreact to negative words; therefore, use positive words, such as "stay calm" instead of negative words, such as "don't fight."

- Stay calm and avoid nervous behavior, such as shuffling your feet, fidgeting, or making abrupt movements.

- Do not restrict the person's movement. If he or she wants to pace, allow it.

- Remain aware that certain acts, such as involving law enforcement, might exacerbate the situation.

- Consider taking a break from the conversation to allow the person a chance to calm down.

Take threats or warnings seriously, particularly if the person believes they are being persecuted. If you are frightened, seek outside help immediately. Never put yourself at risk. Similarly, if the person's aggression escalates out of control at any time, remove yourself from the situation and call for emergency assistance.

If you believe that the aggression is related to a mental health problem, call the mental health crisis team. If you do so, it is best to describe the person's symptoms and behaviors rather than trying to make a diagnosis. Be aware that the crisis team may not attend without a law enforcement presence.

If the situation becomes unsafe, it may be necessary to involve law enforcement. If you suspect the person's aggression is related to a mental health problem, tell law enforcement that you need their help to obtain medical or mental health responders.

Aggressive behavior is frequently associated with intoxication with alcohol or another drug. If you call law enforcement, tell them if the person is intoxicated and what substances you believe have been used.

In either case, tell law enforcement if the person is armed or unarmed.

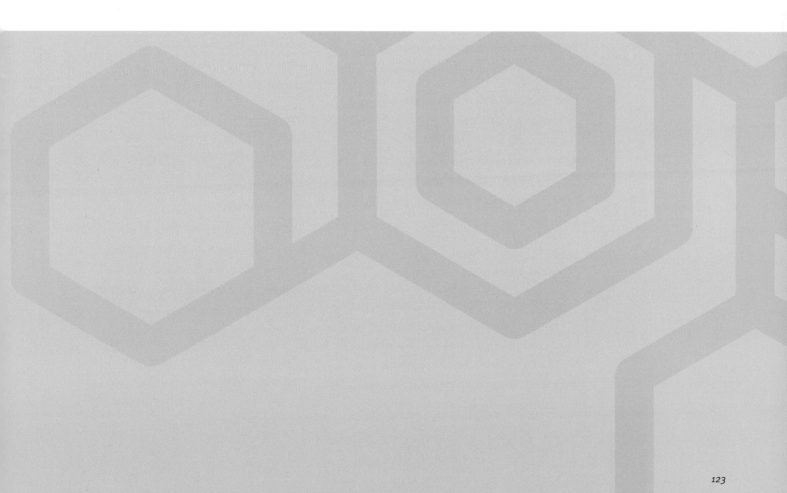

REFERENCES

Foreword

1   *12-Month Prevalence Estimates in the National Comorbidity Survey Replication (NCS-R)*. Harvard School of Medicine, 17 July 2007. Web. 27 Feb. 2013. ‹http://www.hcp.med.harvard.edu/ncs/ftpdir/NCS-R_12-month_Prevalence_Estimates.pdf›.

2   Kessler, R. C., Berglund, P. A., Demler, O., Jin R. and Walters, E. E. (2005) Lifetime prevalence and age-of-onset distributions of DSM-IV Disorders in the National Comorbidity Survey Replication (NCS-R). *Archives of General Psychiatry*. 62, 593-602.

3   Substance Abuse and Mental Health Services Administration, *Results from the 2011 National Survey on Drug Use and Health: Mental Health Findings*, NSDUH Series H-45, HHS Publication No. (SMA) 12-4725. Rockville, MD: Substance Abuse and Mental Health Services Administration, 2012.

4   New Freedom Commission on Mental Health (2003) *Achieving the Promise: Transforming Mental Health Care in America. Final Report* (DHHS Pub. No. SMA-03-3832). Rockville, MD. www.mentalhealthcommission.gov accessed November 3, 2008.

115 Babic, D. (2010). Stigma and mental illness. *Materia Socio Medica*, 22(1), 43-46

5   Teplin, L. A., McClelland, G. M., Abram, K. M., & Weiner, D. A. (2005). Crime victimization in adults with severe mental illness: Comparison with the national crime victimization survey. *Archives of General Psychiatry, 62*, 911-921.

6   Teasdale, B. (2009). Mental disorder and violent victimization. *Criminal Justice and Behavior, 36*(5), 513-535.

7   Frankl, V. (1959) *Man's Search for Meaning. Boston* Beacon, Boston, MA.

8   U.S. Department of Veteran Affairs (n.d.) Suicide prevention. www.mentalhealth.va.gov accessed December 15, 2008.

9   Veterans for Common Sense (n.d.) www.veteransforcommonsense.org accessed December 15, 2008.

10 CBS News (2007): Suicide epidemic among veterans. www.cbsnews.com/stories/2007/11/13/cbsnews_investigates/main3496471.shtml accessed December 15, 2008.

11 Prevention and recovery fact sheet American Psychiatric Association (2012) *Prevention and Recovery*. http://www.psychiatry.org/mental-health/more-topics/national-recovery-month

12 Gagne, C., White, W., & Anthony, W. A. (2007). Recovery: A common vision for the fields of mental health and addictions. *Psychiatric Rehabilitation Journal*, 31(1), 32-37.

13 LeVine, S.E. (2012) Facilitating recovery for people with serious mental illness employing a psychobiosocial model of care. *Professional Psychology: Research and Practice*, 43 (1), 58-64.

14 Pistrang, N., Barker, C. and Humphreys, K. (2008) Mutual help groups for mental health problems: a review of effectiveness studies. *American Journal of Community Psychology*. 42, 110-121.

15 Chien, W. T. , Thompson, D. R., and Norman, I. (2008) Evaluation of a peer-led mutual support group for Chinese families of people with schizophrenia. *American Journal of Community Psychology*. A2, 122-134.

16 University of California (n.d.) Listening first aid. www.cnr.berkeley.edu/ucce50/ag-labor/7article/article40.htm accessed December 16, 2008.

17 Copeland, M. E. (2002) *Wellness Recovery Action Plan*. Peach Press, West Dummerston, VT. Swarbrick, M. (2006) A wellness approach. *Journal of Psychiatric Rehabilitation*. 29, 311-314.

18 Swarbrick, M. (2006). A wellness approach. *Psychiatric Rehabilitation Journal, 4*, 311-313.

19 U.S. Department of Health and Human Services (2008) Question 1: Is there an association between physical activity and depression? www.health.gov/paguidelines/Report/G8_mentalhealth.aspx#_Toc197778613 accessed December 16, 2008.

Chapter 1: Mental Health Problems in the United States

20 World Health Organization (2007) *Mental Health: Strengthening Mental Health Promotion* (Fact Sheet No 220). www.who.int/mediacentre/factsheets/fs220/en/print.html accessed November 3, 2008.

21 American Psychiatric Association (2000) *Diagnostic and Statistical Manual of Mental Disorders, Fourth Edition, Text Revision (DSM-IV-TR)*. Washington, DC.

22 Hudson J. I., Hiripi, E., Pope, H. G. and Kessler, R. C. (2007) The prevalence and correlates of eating disorders in the National Comorbidity Survey Replication. *Biological Psychiatry*. 61, 348-358.

23 Tandon, R., Keshavan, M. S., & Nasrallah, H. A. (2008). Schizophrenia, "just the facts" what we know in 2008. *Schizophrenia Research, 102*, 1-18.

24 World Health Organization. (2008). Disease incidence, prevalence and disability. In World health organization (Ed.), *The Global Burden of Disease: 2004 Update*. Geneva, Switzerland: World Health Organization. Retrieved from http://www.who.int/healthinfo/global_burden_disease/2004_report_update/en/index.html

25 Mathers, C., Boerma, T. and Ma Fat, D. (2008) *The Global Burden of Disease: 2004 Update*. World Health Organization, Geneva, Switzerland. www.who.int/healthinfo/global_burden_disease/GBD_report_2004update/en/index.html accessed November 3, 2008.

26 World Health Organization (2005) *Disease and Injury Regional Estimates for 2004*. www.who.int/healthinfo/global_burden_disease/estimates_regional/en/index.html accessed November 3, 2008.

27 Marshall, M., Lewis, S., Lockwood, A., Drake, R., Jones, P. and Croudace, T. (2005) Association between duration of untreated psychosis and outcome in cohorts of first-episode patients: a systematic review. *Archives of General Psychiatry*. 62, 975-983.

28 Jorm, A. F. (2011). Mental health literacy: Empowering the community to take action for better mental health. *American Psychologist, 67*(3), 231-243.

Chapter 2: Mental Health First Aid

29   ibid.

30   Wang, P. S., Lane, M., Olfson, M., Pincus, H. A., Wells, K. B. and Kessler, R. C. (2005) Twelve-month use of mental health services in the United State: results from the National Comorbidity Survey Replication. *Archives of General Psychiatry.* 62, 629-640.

31   Wang, P. S., Berglund, P., Olfson, M., Pincus, H. A., Wells, K. B. and Kessler, R. C. (2005) Failure and delay in initial treatment contact after first onset of mental disorders in the National Comorbidity Survey Replication. *Archives of General Psychiatry.* 62, 603-613.

Chapter 3: Depression

32   Monroe, S.M., Harkness, K.L. (2011) Recurrence in major depression: A conceptual analysis. *Psychological Review.* Advance online publication. doi:10.1037/a0025190

33   Canuso, C. M., Bossie, C. A., Zhu, Y., Youssef, E. and Dunner, D. L. (2008) Psychotic symptoms in patients with bipolar mania. *Journal of Affective Disorders.* 111, 164-169.

34   Forty, L., Smith, D., Jones, L. et al. (2008) Clinical differences between bipolar and unipolar depression. *British Journal of Psychiatry.* 192, 388-389.

35   Vesga-Lopez, O., Blanco, C., Keyes, K., Olfson, M., Grant, B. F. and Hasin, D. S. (2008) Psychiatric disorders in pregnant and postpartum women in the United States. *Archives of General Psychiatry.* 65, 805-815.

36   Poobalan, A. S., Aucott, L. S., Ross, L., Smith, W. C., Helms, P. J. and Williams, J. H. (2007) Effects of treating postnatal depression on mother-infant interaction and child development: systematic review. *British Journal of Psychiatry.* 191, 378-386.

37   Langlands, R. L., Jorm, A. F., Kelly, C. M. and Kitchener, B. A. (2008) First aid for depression: a Delphi consensus study with consumers, carers and clinicians. *Journal of Affective Disorders.* 105, 157-165.

38   Kelly, C. M. Jorm, A. F., Kitchener, B. A. and Langlands, R. L. (2008) Development of mental health first aid guidelines for suicidal ideation and behaviour: a Delphi study. *BMC Psychiatry.* 8, 17.

39   Borges, G., Angst, J., Nock, M. K., Ruscio, A. M., Walters, E. E. and Kessler, R. C. (2006) A risk index for 12-month suicide attempts in the National Comorbidity Survey Replication (NCS-R). *Psychological Medicine 36.* 1747-1757.

40   National Center for Injury Prevention and Control (2007) *Suicide Facts at a Glance.* Centers for Disease Control and Prevention, Atlanta, GA.

41   Centers for Disease Control and Prevention (2005) *Web-based Injury Statistics Query and Reporting System (WISQARS)* [Online]. Available from www.cdc.gov/ncipc/wisqars/index.htm accessed November 3, 2008.

42   Centers for Disease Control and Prevention (2007) Youth Risk Behavior Surveillance—United States, 2007. Surveillance Summaries, June 6. *MMWR.* 57(No. SS-4).

43 Karch, D., Crosby, A. and Simon, T. (2006) Toxicology testing and results for suicide victims—13 states, 2004. *MMWR.* 55, 1245-1248.

44 Arsenault-Lapierre, G., Kim, C. and Tureck, G. (2004) Psychiatric diagnoses in 3275 suicides: a meta-analysis. *BMC Psychiatry.* 4, 37.

45 Rudd, M. D., Berman, A., Joiner, T. E. et al. (2006) Warning signs for suicide: theory, research and clinical applications. *Suicide and Life-Threatening Behavior.* 36, 255-262.

46 Whitlock, J., Eckenrode, J. and Silverman, D. (2006) Self-injurious behaviors in a college population. *Pediatrics.* 117, 1939-1948.

47 Laye-Gindhu, A. and Schonert-Rechl, K. A. (2005) Nonsuicidal self-harm among community adolescents: understanding the "whats" and "whys" of self-harm. *Journal of Youth and Adolescence.* 4, 447-457.

48 Hawton, K. and James, A. (2005) Suicide and deliberate self harm in young people. *British Medical Journal.* 330, 891-894.

49 Heilbron, N. & Prinstein, M. J. (2008) Peer influence and adolescent nonsuicidal self-injury: a theoretical review of mechanisms and moderators. *Applied and Preventive Psychology.* 12, 169-177.

50 Royal Australian and New Zealand College of Psychiatrists Clinical Practice Guidelines Team for Depression (2004) Australian and New Zealand clinical practice guidelines for the treatment of depression. *Australian and New Zealand Journal of Psychiatry.* 38, 389-407.

51 Cochrane Collaboration Review www.cochrane.org/reviews/en/ab005652.html accessed December 30, 2008.

52 Nasser, E. H., & Overholser, J. C. (2005). Recovery from major depression: The role of support from family, friends, and spiritual beliefs. *Acta Psychiatrica Scandinavica, 111,* 125-132.

116 Krull, E. (2012). Social Support Is Critical for Depression Recovery. *Psych Central.* Retrieved on February 4, 2013, from http://psychcentral.com/lib/2012/social-support-is-critical-for-depression-recovery/

53 Lankappa, S., & Spence, S. A. (2005). Psychiatric in-patients receive fewer greetings cards than other in-patients. *Psychiatric Bulletin, 29,* 449-451.

54 Morgan, A. J. and Jorm, A. F. (2008) Self-help interventions for depressive disorders and depressive symptoms; a systematic review. *Annals of General Psychiatry.* 7, 13.

55 Parker, G. and Crawford, J. (2007) Judged effectiveness of differing antidepressant strategies by those with clinical depression. *Australia and New Zealand Journal of Psychiatry.* 41, 32-37.

56 Christensen, H., Griffiths, K. M. and Jorm, A. F. (2004) Delivering interventions for depression by using the Internet: randomized controlled trial. *British Medical Journal.* 328, 265.

Chapter 4: Anxiety

57 Kessler, R. C., Chiu, W. T., Jin, R., Ruscio, A. M., Shear, K., Walters, E. E. (2006) The epidemiology of panic attacks, panic disorder, and agoraphobia in the National Comorbidity Survey Replication. *Archives of General Psychiatry.* 63, 415-424.

58 Campbell, L. A., Brown, T. A., & Grisham, J. R. (2003). The relevance of age of onset to the psychopathology of generalized anxiety disorder. *Behavior Therapy,* 34, 31-48.

59 Mental Health First Aid Training and Research Program (2008) *Traumatic Events: First Aid Guidelines for Assisting Adults.* ORYGEN Research Centre, University of Melbourne, Australia. www.mhfa.com.au/Guidelines.shtml accessed December 16, 2008.

60 Canadian Psychiatric Association (2006) Clinical practice guidelines: management of anxiety disorders: 2. principles of diagnosis and management of anxiety disorders. *Canadian Journal of Psychiatry.* 51 (Supplement 2), 9S-21S.

61 Jorm, A. F., Christensen, H., Griffiths, K. M., Parslow, R. A., Rodgers, B. and Blewitt, K. A. (2004) Effectiveness of complementary and self-help treatments for anxiety disorders. *Medical Journal of Australia.* 7 (Suppl): S29-46.

62 Manzoni, G. M., Pagnini, F., Castelnuovo, G., and Molinari, E. (2008) Relaxation training for anxiety: a ten-year systematic review with meta-analysis. *BMC Psychiatry.* 2, 41.

Chapter 5: Psychosis

63 Edwards, J. and McGorry, P. D. (2002) *Implementing Early Intervention in Psychosis.* Martin Dunitz, London.

64 Tandon, R., Keshavan, M. S., & Nasrallah, H. A. (2008). Schizophrenia, "just the facts" what we know in 2008. *Schizophrenia Research*, 102, 1-18.

65 McGrath, J., Saha, S., Welham, J., El Saadi, O., MacCauley, C. & Chant, D. (2004) A systematic review of the incidence of schizophrenia: the distribution of rates and the influence of sex, urbanicity, migrant status and methodology. *BMC Medicine.* 2, 13.

66 Robinson, D. G., Woerner, M. G., McMeniman, M., Mendelowitz, A., & Bilder, R. M. (2004). Symptomatic and functional recovery from a first episode of schizophrenia or schizoaffective disorder. *The American Journal of Psychiatry, 161*(3), 473-479.

67 Müller-Oerlinghausen, B., Berghöfer, A. & Bauer, M. (2002) Bipolar disorder. *Lancet.* 359: 241-247.

68 Tandon, R., Keshaven, M. S. and Nasrallah, H. A. (2008) Schizophrenia, "just the facts": what we know in 2008 part 1: epidemiology and etiology. *Schizophrenia Research.* 102, 1-18.

69 Arseneault, L., Cannon, M., Witton, J. and Murray, R. M. (2004) Causal association between cannabis and psychosis: examination of the evidence. *British Journal of Psychiatry.* 184, 110-117.

70 Di Forti, M., Lappin, J. M.and Murray, R. M. (2007) Risk factors for schizophrenia—all roads lead to dopamine. *European Neuropsychopharmacology.* 17 (Suppl 2), S101-107.

71 Tsuchiya, K. J., Byrne, M. and Mortensen, P. B. (2003) Risk factors in relation to an emergence of bipolar disorder: a systematic review. *Bipolar Disorders.* 5, 231-242.

72 Smoller, J. W. and Fin, C. T. (2003) Family, twin, and adoption studies of bipolar disorder. *American Journal of Medical Genetics Part C (Seminars in Medical Genetics)*, 123C, 48-58.

73 Langlands, R. L., Jorm, A. F., Kelly, C. M. and Kitchener, B. A. (2008) First aid recommendations for psychosis: using the Delphi method to gain consensus between mental health consumers, carers, and clinicians. *Schizophrenia Bulletin*. 34, 435-443.

74 ORYGEN Youth Health (2004) *The acute phase of early psychosis: a handbook on management*. ORYGEN Research Centre, *Melbourne, Australia*.

75 Palmer, B. A., Pankratz, V. S. and Bostwick, J. M. (2005) The lifetime risk of suicide in schizophrenia: a reexamination. *Archives of General Psychiatry*. 62, 247-253.

76 Hawton, K., Sutton, L., Haw, C., Sinclair, J. & Deeks, J. J. (2005) Schizophrenia and suicide: systematic review of risk factors. *British Journal of Psychiatry*. 187, 9-20.

77 Fountoulakis, K. N., Gonda, X., Siamouli, M., & Rihmer, Z. (2009). Psychotherapeutic intervention and suicide risk reduction in bipolar disorder: A review of the evidence. *Journal of Affective Disorders, 113*, 21-29.

78 *Violence and Mental Illness: The facts*. (2008, October 24). Retrieved from http://www. stopstigma.samhsa.gov/publications/facts. aspx?printid=1&

79 Friedman, R. A. (2006). Violence and mental illness: How strong is the link?. *The New England Journal of Medicine, 355*(20).

80 ibid.

81 Silver, E. (2006). Understanding the relationship between mental disorder and violence: The need for a criminological perspective. *Law and Human Behavior, 30*(6), 685-706.

82 Tandon, R., Keshaven, M. S. and Nasrallah, H. A. (2008) Schizophrenia, "just the facts": what we know in 2008 part 1: overview. *Schizophrenia Research*. 100, 4-19.

83 McGorry, P., Killackey, E., Elkins, K., Lambert, M. and Lambert, T. (2003) Summary Australian and New Zealand clinical practice guideline's for the treatment of schizophrenia. *Australian Psychiatry*. 11, 136-147.

84 Yatham, L. N., Kennedy, S. H., O'Donovan, C. et al. (2005) Canadian Network for Mood and Anxiety Treatments (CANMAT) guidelines for the management of patients with bipolar disorder: consensus and controversies. *Bipolar Disorders*. 7 (Supplement 3), 5-69.

85 Harrison, I., Joyce, E. M., Mutsatsa, S. H., Hutton, S. B., Huddy, V., Kapasi, M., & Barnes, T. R. E. (2008). Naturalistic follow-up of co-morbid substance use in schizophrenia: the West London first-episode study. *Psychological Medicine, 38*, 79-88.

Chapter 6: Substance Use Disorders

86 Grant, B. F., Stinson, F. S., Dawson, D. A., Chou, P., Duford, M.C., Compton, W. et al. (2004) Prevalence and co-occurrence of substance use disorders and independent mood and anxiety disorders: results from the National Epidemiologic Survey on Alcohol and Related Conditions. *Archives of General Psychiatry*. 61, 807-816.

87 National Institute on Alcohol Abuse and Alcoholism. *U.S. Adult Drinking Patterns*. Excerpted from NIH publication No. 07-3769. www.niaaa.nih.gov/ NR/rdonlyres/E170A639-B684-41A6-8EB6-1237 AF74E56C/o/DrinkingPatterns.pdf accessed December 16, 2008.

88 National Institute on Alcohol Abuse and Alcoholism. *What's a Standard Drink?* Excerpted from NIH publication No. 07-3769. http://pubs.niaaa.nih.gov/publications/tips/tips.pdf accessed November 25, 2008.

89 Cherpitel, C. J. (2002) Screening for alcohol problems in the U.S. general population: comparison of the CAGE, RAPS4, and RAPS4-QF by gender, ethnicity and service utilization. *Alcoholism: Clinical and Experimental Research.* 26, 1686-1691.

90 Center for Behavioral Health Statistics and Quality. (2012). *Results from the 2011 National Survey on Drug Use and Health: Summary of National Findings* (HHS Publication No. SMA 12-4713, NSDUH Series H-44). Rockville, MD: Substance Abuse and Mental Health Services Administration.

91 Substance Abuse and Mental Health Services Administration (2002) *Results from the 2001 National Household Survey on Drug Abuse: Volume I. Summary of National Findings* (Office of Applied Studies, NHSDA Series H-17 ed. BKD461, SMA 02-3758. Washington, DC. www.oas.samhsa.gov/nhsda/2k1nhsda/vol1/Chapter2.htm accessed November 25, 2008.

92 de Win, M. M., Jager, G., Booij, J. et al. (2008) Neurotoxic effects of ecstasy on the thalamus. *British Journal of Psychiatry.* 193: 289-296.

93 Morris, C. D., Waxmonsky, J. A., May, M. G., & Giese, A. A. (2009). What do persons with mental illnesses need to quit smoking? Mental health consumer and provider perspectives. *Psychiatric Rehabilitation Journal, 32*(4), 276-284.

94 Kumari, V., & Postma, P. (2005). Nicotine use in schizophrenia: The self medication hypotheses. *Neuroscience and Biobehavioral Reviews, 29,* 1021-1034.

95 Mental Health First Aid Training and Research Program (2008) *First Aid Guidelines for Problem Drinking.* ORYGEN Research Centre, University of Melbourne, Australia.

96 Gold, M. (2006). Stages of Change. *Psych Central.* Retrieved on December 7, 2012, from http://psychcentral.com/lib/2006/stages-of-change/

97 Willenbring, M. L., Massey, S. H., & Gardner, M. B. (2009). Helping patients who drink too much: An evidence-based guide for primary care physicians. *American Family Physician, 80*(1), 44-50.

98 Moos, R. H. (2007) Theory-based processes that promote the remission of substance use disorders. *Clinical Psychology Review.* 27, 537-551.

Chapter 7: Eating Disorders

99 Hudson, J. I., Hiripi, E., Pope, H. G. and Kessler, R. C. (2007) The prevalence and correlates of eating disorders in the National Comorbidity Survey Replication. *Biological Psychiatry.* 61, 348-358.

100 Mental Health First Aid Training and Research Program (2008) *Eating Disorders: First Aid Guidelines.* ORYGEN Research Centre, University of Melbourne, Australia.

101 Hill, L. S., Reid, F., Morgan, J. F., & Lacey, J. H. (2010). Scoff, the development of an eating disorder screening questionnaire. *International Journal of Eating Disorders, 43*, 344-351.

102 Patton, G. C., Coffey, C. and Sawyer, S. M. (2003) The outcome of adolescent eating disorders: findings from the Victorian Adolescent Health Cohort Study. *European Child and Adolescent Psychiatry*. 12 (Suppl 1), 125-129.

103 National Institute of Mental Health (2007) *Eating Disorders* NIH publication no. 07-4901. U.S. Department of Human Services. National Institutes of Health, Bethesda, MD.

104 Fairburn, C. G. and Harrison, P. J. (2003) Eating disorders. *Lancet*. 361, 407-416.

105 Wilson, G. T., Grilo, C. M. and Vitousek, K. M. (2007) Psychological treatment of eating disorders. *American Psychologist*. 62, 199-216.

106 Perkins, S. J., Murphy, R., Schmidt, U. and Williams, C. (2006) Self-help and guided self-help for eating disorders. *Cochrane Database of Systematic Reviews*. 3, CD004191.

SECTION THREE: FIRST AID FOR MENTAL HEALTH CRISES

First Aid for Suicide

107 Mental Health First Aid Training and Research Program (2008) *Suicidal Thoughts & Behaviors: First Aid Guidelines*. ORYGEN Research Centre, University of Melbourne, Australia. www.mhfa.com.au/Guidelines.shtml accessed December 15, 2008.

First Aid for Nonsuicidal Self-Injury

108 Kelly, C. M., Jorm, A. F., Kitchener, B. A. and Langlands, R. L. (2008) Development of mental health first aid guidelines for nonsuicidal self-injury: a Delphi study. *BMC Psychiatry*. 8, 62.

109 Mental Health First Aid Training and Research Program (2008) *Deliberate Nonsuicidal Self-Injury: First Aid Guidelines*. ORYGEN Research Centre, University of Melbourne, Australia. www.mhfa.com.au/Guidelines.shtml accessed December 16, 2008.

First Aid for Panic Attacks

110 Mental Health First Aid Training and Research Program (2008) *Panic Attacks: First Aid Guidelines*. ORYGEN Research Centre, University of Melbourne, Australia. www.mhfa.com.au/Guidelines.shtml accessed December 16, 2008.

117 Bergeron, J. David; Le Baudour, Chris (2009). "Chapter 9: Caring for Medical Emergencies". *First Responder* (8th ed.). New Jersey: Pearson Prentice Hall. p. 262

First Aid for Adults Affected by Traumatic Events

111 Mental Health First Aid Training and Research Program (2008) *Traumatic Events: First Aid Guidelines for Assisting Adults*. ORYGEN Research Centre, University of Melbourne, Australia. 2008 www.mhfa.com.au/Guidelines.shtml accessed December 16, 2008.

First Aid for Children Affected by Traumatic Events

112 Mental Health First Aid Training and Research Program (2008) *Traumatic Events: First Aid Guidelines for Assisting Children*. ORYGEN Research Centre, University of Melbourne, Australia. www.mhfa.com.au/ Guidelines.shtml accessed December 16, 2008.

First Aid for Acute Psychosis

113 Mental Health First Aid Training and Research Program (2008) *Psychosis: First Aid Guidelines*. ORYGEN Research Centre, University of Melbourne, Australia. www.mhfa.com.au/Guidelines.shtml accessed December 16, 2008.

First Aid for a Medical Emergency from Alcohol Abuse

114 Mental Health First Aid Training and Research Program (2008) *Problem Drinking: First Aid Guidelines*. ORYGEN Research Centre, University of Melbourne, Australia. www.mhfa.com.au/Guidelines. shtml accessed December 16, 2008.

118 The Harvard Medical School Family Health Guide. Recovery Position: Adult Recovery Position. https://www.health.harvard. edu/fhg/firstaid/recovery.shtml accessed March 27, 2013.